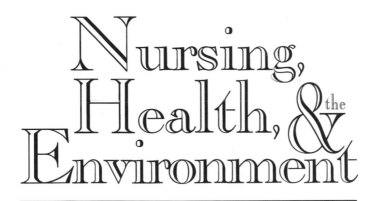

# Nursing, Health, & the Environment

## Strengthening the Relationship to Improve the Public's Health

Andrew M. Pope, Meta A. Snyder, and Lillian H. Mood, Editors

Committee on Enhancing Environmental Health Content
in Nursing Practice

Division of Health Promotion and Disease Prevention

INSTITUTE OF MEDICINE

NATIONAL ACADEMY PRESS
Washington, D.C. 1995

**National Academy Press** • 2101 Constitution Avenue, N.W. • Washington, D.C. 20418

NOTICE: The project that is the subject of this report was approved by the Governing Board of the National Research Council, whose members are drawn from the councils of the National Academy of Sciences, the National Academy of Engineering, and the Institute of Medicine. The members of the committee responsible for the report were chosen for their special competencies and with regard for appropriate balance.

This report has been reviewed by a group other than the authors according to procedures approved by a Report Review Committee consisting of members of the National Academy of Sciences, the National Academy of Engineering, and the Institute of Medicine.

The Institute of Medicine was chartered in 1970 by the National Academy of Sciences to enlist distinguished members of the appropriate professions in the examination of policy matters pertaining to the health of the public. In this, the Institute acts under both the Academy's 1863 congressional charter responsibility to be an adviser to the federal government and its own initiative in identifying issues of medical care, research, and education. Dr. Kenneth I. Shine is President of the Institute of Medicine.

This project was supported by funds from the Agency for Toxic Substances and Disease Registry, the National Institute for Occupational Safety and Health, National Institute of Nursing Research, National Institute of Environmental Health Sciences, Health Resources and Services Administration, and the Environmental Protection Agency (contract number U61/ATU398777-01).

**Library of Congress Cataloging-in-Publication Data**

Nursing, health, and the environment : strengthening the relationship
    to improve the public's health / Andrew M. Pope, Meta A. Snyder, and
    Lillian H. Mood, editors ; Committee on Enhancing Environmental
    Health Content in Nursing Practice, Division of Health Promotion and
    Disease Prevention, Institute of Medicine.
        p.  cm
    Includes bibliographical references and index.
    ISBN 0-309-05298-X
      1. Environmental health. 2. Nursing. 3. Industrial nursing.
    I. Pope, Andrew Mac Pherson, 1950- . II. Snyder, Meta A.
    III. Mood, Lillian H. IV. Institute of Medicine (U.S.). Committee
    on Enhancing Environmental Health Content in Nursing Practice.
      (DNLM: 1. Environmental Health—nurses' instruction.
    2. Environmental exposure—nurses' instruction. 3. Occupational
    Health—nurses' instruction. 4. Nursing. WA 30 N974 1995]
    RA566.N87   1995
    610.73—dc20
    DNLM/DLC
    for Library of Congress                                    95-39601
                                                                 CIP

The serpent has been a symbol of long life, healing, and knowledge among almost all cultures and religions since the beginning of recorded history. The image adopted as a logotype by the Institute of Medicine is based on a relief carving from ancient Greece, now held by the Staatlichemuseen in Berlin.

*Cover photograph*: 1910. Courtesy of Visiting Nurse Service of New York.

## Study Staff

Andrew M. Pope, Study Director
Carrie E. Ingalls, Research Assistant
Michael A. Stoto, Director, Division of Health Promotion and Disease Prevention
Donna Thompson, Administrative Associate
Mona Brinegar, Financial Assistant
Laura Baird, Librarian

# Preface

In this time of local and global environmental concerns, people—as individuals and communities—look increasingly to the health care system for information and advice on identifying and reducing health risks associated with environmental (including workplace) exposure to potential hazards, and for diagnosis and treatment of the diseases caused by such exposures. Nurses are often the first point of contact for patients and concerned individuals, and are in positions to provide considerable support. However, most nurses have little, if any, formal preparation in the field of environmental health.

In response to a growing awareness of the need to enhance occupational and environmental health content in the practice of nursing, a workshop was conducted by the Institute of Medicine (IOM) in May 1993 to assess the need for an IOM study on the role of nurses in occupational and environmental health and to clarify the associated areas of education, training, and research that such a study would involve. It was an illuminating and successful workshop, chaired by Bonnie Rogers, that provided resounding affirmation of the need for the IOM to conduct a full-scale study of issues related to enhancing environmental health content in the practice of nursing.

Following the workshop, and at the request of a consortium of federal agencies, the IOM established the Committee on Enhancing Environmental Health Content in Nursing Practice to carry out the study. Working from the premise that the environment, including the work environment, is a fundamentally important factor in determining the health of individuals and populations, the committee defined essential competencies and curriculum content in environmental health; recommended methods for developing nursing faculty expertise in environmental health; developed strategies for enhancing the dissemination and integration of environmental health content in nursing practice; and identified research issues that would benefit from study by a combination of environmental health and nursing investigators.

I have been privileged to chair the study committee; it is comprised of an amazing group of experts in nursing and environmental practice, education, and research, encompassing a variety of disciplines and diverse perspectives. We particularly benefitted from a deliberate overlap in membership with the IOM Committee on Curriculum Development in Environmental Medicine, which had similar objectives to ours, that is, enhancing environmental health in health care delivery, only with a focus on physicians and medical education.

One of the hallmarks of the committee's work was the mutual respect present among the members. This group's work was an example of true interdisciplinary teamwork—the valuing of differences, openness to others' ideas, a willingness to explore all options, an absence of jockeying for position or recognition, and a generous giving of time, effort, and plain hard work.

The committee met several times during the course of a year, beginning in May 1994, and worked hard at both identifying and resolving issues, and at writing, rewriting, and revising segments of the report. We met as a whole and in small groups with individual and group assignments. Our discussions were held face to face and via conference calls, through FAX, and over the internet. We assembled an even wider circle of opinion and expertise than that represented by the committee through focus groups, surveys, guest presentations, commissioned papers, and literature and research reviews.

Three themes emerged in the process of the study:

1. The environment is a primary determinant of health, and environmental health hazards affect all aspects of life and all areas of nursing practice.

2. Nurses are well positioned for addressing environmental health concerns of individuals and communities. Nurses are the largest group of health professionals; they have great variety in their settings and locations of practice; environmental health is a good fit with the values of the nursing profession regarding disease prevention and social justice; and nurses are trusted by the public.

3. There is a need to enhance the emphasis and awareness of environmental threats to the health of populations served by all areas of nursing practice. This will require changes in practice, education, and research.

This study is not an exercise in defining a new nursing specialty. We recognize that experts will be needed to guide the changes described, and ways are suggested to facilitate the development of those experts. We also realize that some nurses will choose to make environmental issues the primary focus of their practice. Our emphasis, however, is on the role that every nurse can and should play in addressing environmental health issues.

The competencies described for nurses are enhancements of content and focus, as well as some new dimensions of nursing practice. The competencies extend, but are continuous with, nurses' existing roles as investigators, educators, and advocates. The committee's report indicates the need for change for all practicing nurses. Change can seem overwhelming, but it can also be a source of new energy and new interest. Through careful investigation and thoughtful consideration, the committee has made recommendations and proposed strategies for accomplishing these goals. It is not our intent to be prescriptive, but rather to stimulate and challenge the thinking and action of all nurses.

Finally, on behalf of the committee I want to acknowledge all of those who assisted us along the way. A list of these people is presented in Appendix H, but in particular I want to thank M. Virginia Ruth, Barbara Sattler, and Meta Snyder (who also served on the committee) for their assistance in both initiating the study and for providing thoughtful input throughout its tenure. In addition, the workshop and focus group participants deserve recognition for helping us clarify our objectives and the current needs in the field of nursing. The sponsors, of course, are appreciated not only for their initiative and financial support, but also for their substantive contributions and guidance. In particular, we thank the following sponsors: from ATSDR, Max Lum, Diane Narkunas, and Donna Orti; from NIEHS, Anne Sassaman; from NINR, Patricia Moritz; from NIOSH, Bernie Kuchinski and Jane Lipscomb; from EPA, Gershon Bergeisen; and from HRSA, Marla Salmon and Moira Shannon. Perhaps most importantly, I want to thank the IOM for taking the initiative to develop this activity, and for the staff's tireless efforts in guiding us through the shoals of committee work, and for making it an enjoyable, valuable experience.

It was a pleasure to work with such competent professionals on a topic of such fundamental importance. I can only hope that our efforts will indeed enhance the environmental health content of nursing practice and thereby enlarge the indispensable contribution that nurses make to the health of the public. Florence Nightingale would be proud.

Lillian H. Mood
*Chair*

# Acronyms

| | |
|---|---|
| AACN | American Association of Colleges of Nursing |
| AAOHN | American Association of Occupational Health Nurses |
| ABOHN | American Board for Occupational Health Nurses |
| ACHNE | Association of Community Health Nurse Educators |
| ANA | American Nurses Association |
| ANCC | American Nurses Credentialing Center |
| AOEC | Association of Occupational and Environmental Clinics |
| APN | advanced practice nurses |
| ATSDR | Agency for Toxic Substances and Disease Registry |
| | |
| BLS | Bureau of Labor Statistics |
| | |
| CAI | Computer-assisted instruction |
| CD-ROM | compact disk read-only memory |
| CDC | Centers for Disease Control and Prevention |
| CFCs | chlorofluorocarbons |
| CPHF | California Public Health Foundation |
| | |
| DHHS | Department of Health and Human Services |
| DoD | Department of Defense |
| | |
| HRSA | Health Resources and Services Administration |
| | |
| ICN | International Council of Nursing |

| | |
|---|---|
| IOM | Institute of Medicine |
| IRB | institutional review board |
| LPN | licensed practical nurse |
| MFS | medical fee schedule |
| NACNEP | National Advisory Council for Nurse Education and Practice |
| NANDA | North American Nursing Diagnosis Association |
| NBCSN | National Boards for Certification of School Nurses |
| NCEH | National Center for Environmental Health |
| NCLEX | National Council Licensure Examination for Registered Nurses |
| NCSBN | National Council of State Boards of Nursing |
| NIEHS | National Institute of Environmental Health Sciences |
| NIJ | National Institute of Justice |
| NINR | National Institute of Nursing Research |
| NIOSH | National Institute for Occupational Safety and Health |
| NLN | National League for Nursing |
| NP | nurse practitioner |
| OSHA | Occupational Safety and Health Administration |
| PPRC | Physician Payment Review Commission |
| RN | registered nurse |
| STTI | Sigma Theta Tau International |
| TRI | Toxic Chemical Release Inventory |

# Contents

*xi*

# Nursing, Health, & the Environment

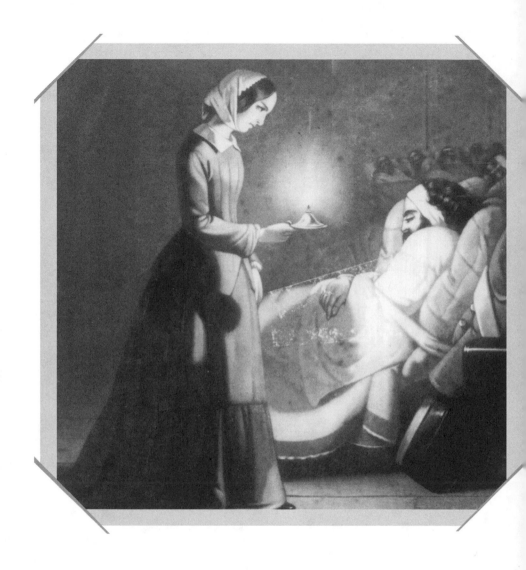

*"An Angel of Mercy." Florence Nightingale
at a soldier's bedside at Scutari.*

# Executive Summary

*Every day sanitary knowledge, or the knowledge of nursing, or in other words, of how to put the constitution in such a state as that it will have no disease, or that it can recover from disease, takes a higher place.*

—Florence Nightingale, 1860, Preface

## ABSTRACT

Environmental health hazards, including those in the work environment, are ubiquitous, often insidious, and generally poorly understood. As such, they are of increasing interest to the general public and of fundamental importance to health care providers.

Among health care providers, registered nurses occupy a unique position. In both rural and urban settings, nurses are often the initial, and sometimes the only, point of contact for people seeking medical care. They are also the largest group of professional health care providers in the United States: an estimated 2.2 million. In occupational health practice, nurses outnumber physicians by six to one. Yet the vast majority of nurses have had no formal training in occupational or environmental health.

If environmental health hazards and health effects are to be recognized and dealt with effectively, it is of fundamental importance that all health care providers have a clear understanding of the association between the environment and health. Toward that end the committee makes a series of recommendations for the integration and enhancement of environmental health in nursing education, practice, and research.

## INTRODUCTION

The environment is one of the primary determinants of individual and community health. And, whether it is justifiable or not, there is

1

growing public concern and apprehension about the potential adverse health effects associated with exposure to substances in the home, the workplace, and in the other community settings. Unfortunately, most health care providers, including nurses, are inadequately prepared to identify or respond appropriately to such hazards or conditions.

A comprehensive approach to nursing practice (as well as other health care professions) requires the awareness, recognition, and treatment of critical factors that affect individual and community health, even if these factors are not obvious at first to patients or providers. A child who has a behavior problem in school because of lead poisoning; a young adult who has respiratory problems due to the inhalation of solvents while working in the garage at home; a worker who is exhibiting neurological symptoms related to handling chemicals on the job; and a retired person whose rash is caused by a garden pesticide are all examples of people who have been affected by environmental health hazards in ways that could easily be misinterpreted in the absence of information about the origin of the problem.

Nurses are well positioned to address environmental health hazards, both on an individual and community level, for a number of reasons: They are the largest group of health care providers in the United States (2.2 million), and generally speaking, they have more opportunities than other health care providers to talk in-depth with patients. In addition, they are often the only health care providers who visit patients in their homes, workplaces, and local communities, thus gaining firsthand knowledge of the potential environmental hazards present in these settings. The close interaction of nurses with patients and the "on-site" aspects of nursing care provide tremendous opportunities for nurses to detect previously unrecognized health problems, including those related to environmental exposures, and to initiate appropriate interventions. Finally, there is a good fit between environmental health concerns, the historical development of the nursing profession, and core nursing values.

## DEFINING ENVIRONMENTAL HEALTH

The committee recognizes a need to distinguish between issues of environmental health and issues more specific to the science of ecology. The primary focus of this report is on the adverse health outcomes that may be associated with exposure to environmental hazards rather than efforts to conserve natural resources. This focus is in no way intended to diminish the importance of ecological issues.

The environmental hazards of concern in this report fall into four widely accepted classes: chemical, physical, biological, and psychosocial. Such hazards may be naturally occurring, such as radon or ultraviolet light from the sun, or they may be manmade (or "constructed"), such as particulates and gases released into the environment from automotive exhaust, industrial sources or tobacco smoke. As these examples demonstrate, environmental hazards may be encountered in the home, workplace, and community environments. Thus, adverse health outcomes related to environmental conditions include worker and childhood lead poisoning, childhood and occupationally induced asthma, and repetitive motion injury, among many others. Taken in this context, use of the term *environmental health* throughout this report refers to freedom from illness or injury related to exposure to toxic agents and other environmental conditions that are potentially detrimental to human health.

## ENVIRONMENTAL HEALTH HAZARDS

Since 1950, more than 65,000 new chemical compounds have been introduced into common use in the western world, the majority of which (84 percent) have not been tested for human toxicity. The post-World War II era brought major technological advances that were accompanied by the release of an unprecedented number of new synthetic chemicals onto United States markets. New chemical compounds continue to be introduced into the environment each year; presently, 72,000 chemicals are used in commerce in the United States, and most have had limited testing for their effects on human health. Furthermore, the U.S. Environmental Protection Agency (EPA) reports that more than 40 million people live within 4 miles of a Superfund site,[1] and approximately 4 million people reside within 1 mile of a site, further increasing their risk of exposure.

In the home, other environmental hazards have well-documented adverse human health effects. These include radon, environmental tobacco smoke, pesticides, carbon monoxide and airborne particulates from wood-burning stoves, nitrogen dioxide from natural gas stoves, formaldehyde and other chemicals that are released as "off-gases" from new carpets, blown-in foam insulation, and the synthetic materials that cover the indoor surfaces of many mobile homes.

Environmental hazards in occupational settings can be substantial, and workplace injuries and fatalities are the best-documented environmental effects on health. More than 2.25 million work-related illnesses

---

[1]Superfund sites are hazardous waste sites designated by the EPA to be a threat to human health; these may include leaking underground storage tanks or inactive hazardous waste sites such as municipal dumps and contaminated factories or mines and mills (Chiras, 1994, p. 462).

and injuries were reported to the U.S. Department of Labor in 1993, the most recent year for which data are available.

Finally, in addition to community, home, and workplace exposures, global environmental conditions may adversely affect human health. The global warming trends experienced over the last century may have numerous untoward health effects should they continue. For example, it has been estimated that mortality in U.S. cities during prolonged heat waves may increase by 30–50 percent if current warming trends continue. Depletion of stratospheric ozone due to the release of chlorofluorocarbons, which has occurred over the Arctic as well as over the Antarctic, leaves large populations of people in other parts of the world at risk for adverse health effects from overexposure to ultraviolet radiation.

In summary, a large spectrum of environmental agents are potential health hazards. Some of these agents are common, others are not; some are easily detected, others are not. All of these hazards are important, however, and nurses need to be aware of them in their daily practice to improve the level of health care that they provide.

## NURSING PRACTICE

With environmental influences on health so widespread and so consequential, an understanding of environmental health is important in all areas of nursing practice, including assessment, diagnosis, planning, intervention, and evaluation. This is already recognized to a large extent in community and public health nursing and in occupational health nursing. For example, occupational health nurses routinely take environmental influences and concerns into account when assessing a patient's health status. The same approach needs to be used more widely in other areas of nursing practice.

It is not the intent of this committee to encourage the creation of a new environmental health specialty within nursing, particularly because closely related specialties already exist. Rather, the committee supports the importance of increasing environmental health awareness and content for all nurses, regardless of their particular field of practice or educational preparation. There is a fundamental need for the entire nursing community to develop a greater understanding of environmental health hazards and the skills needed to incorporate environmental health into practice. The essential skills include a basic understanding of common environmental and occupational health hazards, prevention and abatement methods, and the resources available for referral and assistance (see Box 1, "General Environmental Health Competencies for Nurses").

If environmental health concerns are to be included in practice in meaningful ways, nurses will need to function as members of profes-

---

**Box 1**
**General Environmental Health Competencies for Nurses**

I. *Basic knowledge and concepts*
  All nurses should understand the scientific principles and underpinnings of the relationship between individuals or populations, and the environment (including the work environment). This understanding includes the basic mechanisms and pathways of exposure to environmental health hazards, basic prevention and control strategies, the interdisciplinary nature of effective interventions, and the role of research.

II. *Assessment and referral*
  All nurses should be able to successfully complete an environmental health history, recognize potential environmental hazards and sentinel illnesses, and make appropriate referrals for conditions with probable environmental etiologies. An essential component of this is the ability to access and provide information to patients and communities, and to locate referral sources.

III. *Advocacy, ethics, and risk communication*
  All nurses should be able to demonstrate knowledge of the role of advocacy (case and class), ethics, and risk communication in patient care and community intervention with respect to the potential adverse effects of the environment on health.

IV. *Legislation and regulation*
  All nurses should understand the policy framework and major pieces of legislation and regulations related to environmental health.

---

sional teams. For effective teamwork, the educational preparation of all health professionals—nurses, physicians, and allied health professionals—need to place a greater emphasis on skills needed for interprofessional collaboration, such as negotiation, critical thinking, and mutual problem solving. In addition, there must be opportunities for interdisciplinary interaction throughout professional education and clinical practice, and existing barriers to interdisciplinary practice must be removed.

Interventions in environmental health problems often require nurses and other health care professionals to assume the roles of advocate, activist, and policy planner on behalf of an individual patient or population of patients. Patient advocacy, bringing a patient's concerns to the attention of the physician within the health care setting, is familiar to most, if not all, nurses. However, advocacy that goes beyond the confines of the health care system is a new kind of activity for many nurses, who may feel ill equipped for translating research and practice issues into health policy terms.

Advocacy that goes beyond helping an individual patient and enters the realm of health policy is not yet acceptable and expected nursing practice for all nurses. To prepare the profession for a broader range of advocacy activities, nursing curriculum and continuing education programs may come to include content on such skills as lobbying, use of the media, mediation, expert testimony, and community organizing. In the meantime, whether with institutional support or on their own, nurses who are stretching the definitional boundaries of advocacy practice will need to build skills in areas that were likely not part of their basic nursing education.

## NURSING EDUCATION

The majority of nurses confronting environmental health problems have not received adequate basic preparation to recognize and respond to them, will not attend graduate school, and must rely on continuing education programs to sustain and augment their level of knowledge. A national survey of occupational and environmental health content in baccalaureate nursing schools indicated that only one-third included occupational and environmental health factors as part of routine patient assessment. In addition, in its Seventh Report to the President and the U.S. Congress, the U.S. Department of Health and Human Services noted not only significant shortages of occupational and environmental health personnel but also a serious deficit in nurses' educational preparation concerning basic theories, principles, and methods of public health. Lacking the training and education necessary to recognize the health effects of environmental agents, nurses cannot begin to intervene appropriately to prevent further illnesses, injuries, or fatalities.

Opportunities for nurses to learn about, obtain experience in, and otherwise develop expertise in environmental health are quite limited. Educational resources intended specifically for training nurses in this area are almost nonexistent. There are no nursing texts or professional nursing organizations with a primary focus on environmental health issues, and there are no graduate-level training programs in schools of nursing that focus on environmental health. One indicator of nursing education's lack of emphasis on environmental health is the limited content included in nursing textbooks. Federal support for nursing programs in environmental health is currently limited to a small number of graduate level training programs sponsored by the National Institute for Occupational Safety and Health.

To better prepare nurses for the environmental aspects of nursing practice, the environmental health curriculum content in all levels of nursing education should be enhanced. The committee recognizes that integrating environmental health content into an already crowded curriculum will require creativity on the part of faculty, as well as commitment on the part of educational administrators. Instead of viewing this content as completely new and separate, nursing educators may find ways to emphasize the environmental dimensions of existing courses.

The committee's approach to enhancing education in environmental health was not to develop a new curriculum or to dictate those elements that should be part of basic nursing education. Rather the committee's intent was to help faculty in nursing programs think about and incorporate environmental health content into existing courses (or curricula). To that end, this report deals with four curricular concerns: (1) identifying the general competencies relevant to environmental health in nursing, (2) suggesting where those competencies may be addressed and integrated into the curriculum, (3) providing examples of content areas conducive to the inclusion of environmental health in order to link educational activities with the competencies to be achieved, and (4) suggesting resources that will facilitate the teaching of environmental health issues. A summary of the committee's approach is presented in Table 4.1 in Chapter 4 of the report which lists core courses commonly found in nursing programs. Accompanying each course are the competencies that could be addressed therein, an example of suggested content relevant to the course, and references and resources.

The committee also recognizes that most nurses will continue to be educated at less-than baccalaureate levels, where fewer opportunities exist for including environmental health content. Moreover, nurses already in practice will not benefit directly from curricular changes in basic nursing education. Meeting the environmental health training needs of nurses in associate degree and diploma programs, and of nurses already in practice will require the development of continuing education opportunities and other kinds of professional support. In other words, a range of different strategies will be needed because of the widely varying education and employment circumstances of registered nurses (RNs).

## NURSING RESEARCH

Nursing research is geared to understanding human responses and behavior in regard to health rather than to an elucidation of diseases and their treatment or cure. Clarifying the complex relationship between human behavior and the physical and biological effects of environmental hazards with the goal of facilitating social and behavioral changes is a major focus of nursing research in environmental health. The knowledge generated from nursing research shows how people achieve health, respond to threats to their health, and cope with disease and the treatment of disease. In nursing research the view of people (seen individually or collectively) is holistic, and a priority is the preservation of human autonomy in the achievement of health. Thus, in the area of environmental health, nursing research addresses (1) human responses to potential and real environmental hazards and (2) interventions directed toward the prevention of exposure to environmental hazards (primary intervention), the limitation of exposure to the hazards (secondary intervention), and treatment or rehabilitation after exposure to environmental hazards (tertiary intervention). Nursing research also addresses the quality and safety of the physical environment from the perspective of how people interact with their environment during the course of their daily lives. An example of this type of research is the work-related enhancement of person-environment compatibility through reductions of ambient stresses such as noise levels. Nursing research is also directed toward quality control of the physical environment and related public policy. Nursing research thus spans the area from individual biological (e.g., physical symptoms of lead poisoning) and behavioral (e.g., ingestion of paint chips) responses to environmental hazards, to collective and group behavior (e.g., community efforts or regulatory policy aimed at removing a hazard).

In order to assess the status of research in nursing, a survey of the literature was conducted. The survey showed that there is, in general, a dearth of research in environmental or occupational health related to the practice of nursing. Overall, nursing research represents an extremely small component of the portfolio of funded research of the agencies and organizations polled: 9 of 1,367 (0.6 percent) government grants and 12 of 3,124 (0.4 percent) grants from professional and private research organizations. The reason for this underrepresentation was not explored, but it likely reflects the small number of people conducting nursing research. Thus, nurse researchers and nursing research in the area of environmental or occupational health are underrepresented both in terms of numbers and activity. Further, nonnurse investigators in the area of environmental or occupational health do not appear to be conducting studies directly related to the knowledge base for nursing practice. Expansion of the research directly related to nursing practice in the area of environmental or occupational health is most likely to be accomplished by expanding the level of research conducted by nurse investigators.

Currently, nurse principal investigators in the area of environmental and occupational health identified in the survey are mainly affiliated with schools of nursing (48.6 percent). Interestingly, there is a larger proportion of nurse principal investigators working in corporate settings (20 percent) than in other, nonnursing university units (11.4 percent), such as in schools of public health. This finding most likely reflects the predominant occupational health focus of the studies captured in the literature survey (91.4 percent). Schools of nursing and universities are the administrative homes for the majority of the nurse investigators in environmental or occupational health. However, the private sector is also active in nursing research.

The scope of the research studies surveyed (grants and published papers) was broad in terms of topics, subject groups, and health hazards or conditions studied. In contrast, the type of design and total funding for nursing research appear to be limited. Current nursing research in the area of environmental or occupational health appears to be predominantly descriptive rather than clinical. This is a serious limitation because the application of knowledge to practice generally follows clinical intervention studies. To conduct research that can serve as a basis for clinical nursing practice in environmental or occupational health, it may be necessary to conduct some descriptive studies to identify appropriate and valid biobehavioral models from which nursing interventions could emanate. However, the highly descriptive research found in the survey might also reflect an inadequate focus of the research on clinical intervention strategies for nurses, even though it is conducted by nurse investigators. It is difficult to ascertain information regarding the nurse's role in multidisciplinary team research where the nurse is not a co-investigator.

Regardless of the reason for the predominantly descriptive nature of nursing research, it is clear that scant research supports the clinical practice of nursing in environmental health. Because nursing, like other health professions, strives to base its clinical practice and educational programs on knowledge generated from research, the volume of relevant clinical data in environmental health must be increased to support nursing practice in this area. To generate an adequate knowledge base to support nursing practice in environmental or occupational health, the numbers of nurse researchers and funded projects must be increased, and the design of the work must be broadened to include experimental and intervention studies.

## SUMMARY OF RECOMMENDATIONS

Table 1 contains a listing of all of the recommendations presented in this report. Each recommendation is elaborated on in its respective chapter with a rationale and strategies for implementation.

TABLE 1 Summary listing of all recommendations in this report

### Nursing Practice

**Recommendation 3.1**: Environmental health should be reemphasized in the scope of responsibilities for nursing practice.

**Recommendation 3.2**: Resources to support environmental health content in nursing practice should be identified and made available.

**Recommendation 3.3**: Nurses should participate as members and leaders in interdisciplinary teams that address environmental health problems.

**Recommendation 3.4**: Communication should extend beyond counseling individual patients and families to facilitating the exchange of information on environmental hazards and community responses.

**Recommendation 3.5**: The concept of advocacy in nursing should be expanded to include advocacy on behalf of groups and communities, in addition to advocacy on behalf of individual patients and their families.

**Recommendation 3.6**: Conduct research regarding the ethical implications of occupational and environmental health hazards and incorporate findings into curricula and practice.

### Nursing Education

**Recommendation 4.1**: Environmental health concepts should be incorporated into all levels of nursing education.

**Recommendation 4.2**: Environmental health content should be included in nursing licensure and certification examinations.

**Recommendation 4.3**: Expertise in various environmental health disciplines should be included in the education of nurses.

**Recommendation 4.4**: Environmental health content should be an integral part of lifelong learning and continuing education for nurses.

**Recommendation 4.5**: Professional associations, public agencies, and private organizations should provide more resources and educational opportunities to enhance environmental health in nursing practice.

### Nursing Research

**Recommendation 5.1**: Multidisciplinary and interdisciplinary research endeavors should be developed and implemented to build the knowledge base for nursing practice in environmental health.

**Recommendation 5.2**: The number of nurse researchers should be increased to prepare to build the knowledge base in environmental health as it relates to the practice of nursing.

**Recommendation 5.3**: Research priorities for nursing in environmental health should be established and used by funding agencies for resource allocation decisions and to give direction to nurse researchers.

**Recommendation 5.4**: Current efforts to disseminate research findings to nurses, other health care providers, and the public should be strengthened and expanded.

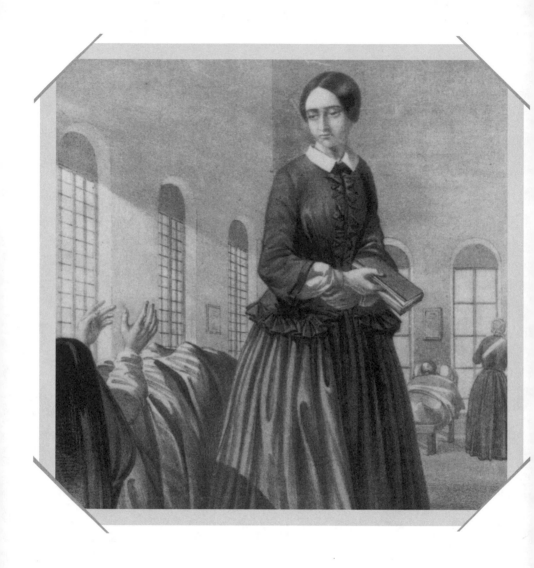

*Portrait of Florence Nightingale in a hospital ward used on the cover of the sheet music for a popular ballad written in her honor, "The Nightingale's Song to the Sick and Wounded."*

# 1

# Introduction

*I use the word nursing for want of a better. It has been limited to signify little more than the administration of medicines and the application of poultices. It ought to signify the proper use of fresh air, light, warmth, cleanliness, quiet, and the proper selection and administration of diet—all at the least expense of vital power to the patient.*

—Florence Nightingale, 1860, p. 8

At its inception, the profession of nursing adopted a holistic approach toward health promotion and the prevention of illness and injury. Florence Nightingale founded modern nursing on the tenet that the role of the nurse was primarily to modify the environment in ways that enhanced health and healing. Her classic text *Notes on Nursing* (Nightingale, 1860), the first volume to codify nursing practice, includes topics such as ventilation and heating, health of houses, noise, light, food, and cleanliness. In Nightingale's view, any factor that can affect the health of the patient and the health of the public was relevant to nursing practice.

At the time that nursing began to emerge as a profession, the interaction of the environment and health was difficult to ignore. Nurses worked predominately in the community, overseeing the care of the sick in homes, work sites, and schools, where environmental threats to health were often extreme and highly visible (DeWitt, 1990; Kalisch and Kalisch, 1986; Moore, 1990; O'Reilly, 1990; Pierson, 1990; Scovil, 1990). In those early days, nursing care included responsibility for "the construction, sanitation, and hygiene of all places where people pass their waking hours or sleep" (Davis, 1990). However, despite the good fit between environmental health concerns, core nursing values, and the profession's early history, over the years environmental factors increasingly came to be treated as separate from the nursing domain. As hospitals assumed a greater role in the health care system, more nurses were employed in noncommunity-based settings (Kalisch and Kalisch, 1986). Nursing care focused increasingly on the individual patient's health, specifically, the treatment of disease and rehabilitation. Less emphasis was placed on preventive care in general, including the elimination of harmful environments and the enhancement of healthful environments.

This trend continues in nursing today. Environmental health currently receives scant attention in nursing education and research (Rogers, 1991, 1994; Snyder et al., 1994). Neither the present organizational structure of nursing practice nor the reimbursement mechanisms presently in place for nurses favor the development of nursing skills related to environmental health hazards. In fact, numerous barriers discourage or prevent nurses from fulfilling their potential in this regard. Environmental health hazards have come to be perceived as something separate from the usual practice of nursing rather than as a set of concerns integral to its mission.

Nevertheless, nurses remain well positioned to address the potential health effects from environmental hazards at both the individual and community levels. The 2.2 million registered nurses in the United States make up the nation's largest group of health care providers (HRSA, 1992). On a daily basis, regardless of specialty or practice site, nurses meet people who are at risk or ill because of hazards in the environment such as contaminated food or drinking water, toxic waste, occupational exposures to harmful substances and conditions, lead and radon in the home, and health-threatening conditions related to poverty. The health benefits to patients from nurses' better education and fuller involvement in addressing environmental health concerns are potentially enormous.

The intent of this report is to remind providers, planners, administrators, observers, and receivers of nursing services that environmental health concerns should not be left to others or relegated to a small group of nursing specialists. On the contrary, these concerns are relevant to the entire nursing community, being part and parcel of the holistic health approach that nursing at its best has always championed.

## DEFINING ENVIRONMENTAL HEALTH

The committee recognizes a need to distinguish between issues of environmental health and issues more specific to the science of ecology. The primary focus of this report is on the adverse health outcomes that may be associated with exposure to environmental hazards rather than efforts to conserve natural resources. This is in no way intended to diminish the importance of ecological issues.

The environmental hazards of concern in this report fall into four widely accepted classes: chemical, physical, biological, and psychosocial. Such hazards may be naturally occurring, such as radon or ultraviolet light from the sun, or they may be manmade (or "constructed"), such as particulates and gases released into the environment from automotive exhaust, industrial sources or tobacco smoke. As these examples demonstrate, environmental hazards may be encountered in the home, workplace, and community environments. Thus, adverse health outcomes related to environmental conditions include worker and childhood lead poisoning, childhood and occupationally induced asthma, and repetitive motion injury, among many others. Taken in this context, use of the term *environmental health* throughout this report refers to freedom from illness or injury related to exposure to toxic agents and other environmental conditions that are potentially detrimental to human health.

The committee includes the workplace in this definition because the workplace is the locus of some of the most significant environmental exposures. Moreover, many concepts and principles from the field of occupational health and occupational health nursing are directly relevant and applicable to broader environmental health issues.

Some health problems that nurses encounter fit easily into the definition of environmental health given above (e.g., lead poisoning). There is heated debate over others that exist in the overlap between health and social problems. For example, interpersonal violence has not been traditionally regarded as an environmental health issue. Some argue that violence is an environmental health problem, because violence represents a major and growing threat to health in the environments of many people (NRC, 1993a). The committee wishes to underscore that all definitions of environmental health are socially constructed, reflecting politics as well as science. Nurses and other health professionals must remember that the conceptual boundaries of environmental health are not set in stone and may expand or narrow as social priorities change and as scientific knowledge increases.

## ENVIRONMENTAL HEALTH AS A CORE FUNCTION OF NURSING PRACTICE

As defined in this report, environmental hazards to human health affect all areas of nursing practice. Nurses, often the first contact point in the health care system and with responsibility for managing the care of individuals over time, are well positioned to ask questions and make observations that can lead to the accurate assessment of and prompt intervention in problems related to environmental conditions and exposures. Pediatric nurses, for example, need to be vigilant with respect to specific hazards for children, such as residential lead paint, and knowledgeable of children's unique vulnerabilities to environmental agents caused by rapid growth and cell division, higher metabolic and respiratory rates, and dietary patterns that differ from those of adults (NRC, 1993b). Gerontology and oncology nurses need to understand that cancers and other diseases in older people may be due in whole or in part to toxic exposures that occurred years earlier in the workplace, home, or community. Nurses working in obstetrics and gynecology need to be aware that many environmental hazards are known to affect adversely reproductive health or are suspected of doing so (Paul, M., 1993). Emergency department and trauma nurses need to know how to isolate, decontaminate, and treat workers and emergency response personnel who are exposed to toxic chemicals through transportation spills, industrial accidents, or unsafe working conditions. Occupational health nurses, who already address health hazards in the work environment, need to be wary of workplace chemicals that can be carried into the community as effluent or into homes on the clothing of workers, putting additional populations at risk.

In particular, any nurse caring for economically disadvantaged patients should be aware that these populations often face an increased risk of exposure to hazardous environmental pollutants. For example, low-income and minority populations are more likely to live near or work in heavily polluting industries, hazardous waste dump sites, and incinerators (EPA, 1992). They are more likely to live in substandard houses with friable asbestos and deteriorating lead paint and to have yards with contaminated soil. They are also more likely to be exposed to toxic chemicals through diets that include seafood or fish taken from local waters designated unfit for swimming and fishing. Thus, the environmental burden is generally greater for minorities and the economically disadvantaged because they are exposed to a greater number and intensity of environmental pollutants in food, air, water, homes, and workplaces. Inequities of this kind have generated sharp controversies, often cast in terms of "environmental justice," about legislative and regulatory measures that can be used to decrease the burden of pollution on disadvantaged communities. The environmental justice issue has special relevance to this report, because for many disadvantaged populations, nurses represent the initial and most consistent point of contact with the health care system. Because of their close contact, nurses are well positioned to represent the environmental concerns of members of these communities in discussions of health policy.

Individuals and communities often lack adequate information about environmental hazards to enable them to act on their own behalf. There are a variety of reasons for this lack of access to information, such as the use of overly technical language in warning signs, illiteracy, and language inadequacies. Nurses are responsible for responding to an individual's or a community's lack of access to information.

## MOVING TO A POPULATION-BASED PERSPECTIVE

At present, when the nursing profession addresses environmental health at all, it is generally in the context of the individual patient or the patient's family. However, as in the case of health issues related to environmental justice, an equally important dimension of environmental health is the community context. Populations of entire neighborhoods and regions can be affected by industrial pollution, waste disposal facilities, contaminated streams and soil, toxic incinerator emissions, and other potential environmental threats to health.

The effects of environmental hazards on the health of the community often generate public controversy, and concerned citizens organize their communities to protect their health, legal, and financial interests. One of the most familiar examples occurred at Love Canal, New York, in the 1960s when citizens learned that their residential neighborhood was contaminated with potentially dangerous industrial waste. They organized under the leadership of Lois Gibbs, a resident of the community with no special training in environmental issues, and sought professional help from local and state health department officials and scientific experts. Their concern eventually grew into a major social movement involving litigation, social protest, and government intervention. Because of the national media attention that the movement received, Love Canal became an important symbol for the national environmental movement. Ms. Gibbs' organization developed its own scientific expertise through self-training with expert assistance. The organization subsequently developed into a national resource center (see Appendix D), offering technical assistance to communities facing environmental health threats. Other more recent examples of community-based environmental health activism abound (Ashford, 1994; Needleman and Landrigan, 1994). Some of these efforts occur on an entirely local level. Others (for example, dioxin in the soil at Times Beach, Missouri, and contaminated drinking water at Woburn, Massachusetts) have been covered intensively by the national press and television networks and have become the focus of major health research efforts.

In such situations, residents of the community tend to seek help from local health professionals, including nurses. Residents will especially turn to nurses working in public health, community health, and occupational health, but nurses outside these specializations may also be drawn into the issue simply because they reside in the area and are trusted by the community. Whether or not they are prepared for the role, nurses in all fields of practice may find themselves interacting with worried residents of the community. They may be asked to assess, advise, and counsel pregnant women who are concerned about the possibility of birth defects, parents concerned about the safety of the drinking water or children's play areas, workers at high risk of cancer from occupational chemical exposures, workers' compensation claimants and community litigants seeking redress for their injuries, and homeowners with questions about the health effects of residential lead or radon, as well as questions about the costs of mitigating the hazard.

In responding to citizen concerns of this kind, most nurses are at a distinct disadvantage, because in general, there is a wide disparity between a public health orientation and the way that nurses are taught to practice their profession. Public health issues must be approached from a population-based, primary prevention perspective. Yet, most nurses practice their profession from a curative perspective that focuses on ill individuals. This mismatch creates conceptual and practical difficulties for nurses involved with environmental health issues. They may feel that they lack the authority to take a public health approach or that they lack the skills to analyze health issues in population-based terms. They may be interested in reconceptualizing the ways in which environmental factors fit into their nursing practice, but they are too pressured and busy to consider such a reconceptualization. In light of the controversy that sometimes surrounds public health issues, nurses may feel safer caring for individuals because this is the task with which they are more familiar; caring for individuals allows nurses to stay solidly within the boundaries of the health care system without stepping into the social, legal, and political arenas important for disease prevention.

Tension between the paradigm of public health and the paradigm of individual care, a serious concern in environmental health, also underlies many other current debates in health care (Barnes et al., 1995). One goal of this report is to provide realistic guidance and assistance to nurses in various practice roles so that they can bridge the gulf between the two frameworks in relation to environmental health.

## THE NURSING WORKFORCE

Preparing nurses to respond more effectively to environmental health problems raises complex professional issues, in part because nursing offers so many different levels of training and routes to practice. The term *nurse* as used in this report refers to *registered nurses* (RNs) who have graduated from an accredited nursing education program and who have passed the licensure examination. However, not all RNs are the same in terms of educational background, clinical experience, or preparation. The entry-level professional licensure examination (NCLEX, National Council Licensure Examination for Registered Nurses) does not include content specific to environmental health or general concepts of population-based practice central to public health, which include the environment as a primary determinant of health. The current curricular content relevant to environmental health varies dramatically among professional nursing education programs.

Despite their common licensure status, not all nurses are trained to practice in the same settings, with the same level of skill, or in the same roles. Most RNs receive their basic nursing education in one of three programs: hospital diploma, associate degree, or baccalaureate degree.[1] Graduates with hospital diplomas and associate degrees are prepared primarily as skilled members of the team that delivers direct patient care services in institutional settings. Nurses with baccalaureate degrees are likewise prepared primarily for patient care in institutional or organized care settings, including community-based health care facilities. However, they also serve in leadership roles and are expected to revise nursing practice, conduct quality control analyses, and participate in research.

Nurses with clinical graduate degrees and/or specialty certification are commonly referred to as advanced practice nurses (APNs). These include clinical nurse specialists, who are often employed in tertiary-care settings, and nurse practitioners, who often work in the community (AACN, 1994). These nurses are prepared for leadership roles in advanced practice and collaborative roles with other health care professionals. Independent practice and practice in partnership with physicians may require educational preparation at the master's level or higher as well as national certification. These nurses structure, implement, and evaluate systems of health care delivery in hospitals or community-based settings and provide continuing education to other staff to improve practice. While some APNs may have received some formal preparation in environmental health concepts through occupational health nursing programs at the master's or doctoral level, the supply of nurses with this kind of training is meager.

One of the fundamental problems related to enhancing environmental health content in nursing practice is the fact that only about one-third of the nurses in community-based settings have formal training in public health or environmental health concepts and the related clinical experience necessary to deal adequately with the environmental aspects of health. This problem has occurred because only nurses prepared at the baccalaureate level or higher are likely to have formal training in basic public health and environmental health concepts, and only one-third of the RNs in community-based settings have training at the baccalaureate

---

[1]A small number of nurses obtain their basic nursing preparation in master's degree programs.

level or higher; the other two-thirds are largely graduates of associate degree programs that provide only an observational experience in community care settings (HRSA, 1992) (see Chapter 4).

This mismatch between the level of educational preparation of RNs and their practice settings and roles in relation to environmental health is part of a more general problem in the composition of the nursing workforce. In a recent review of priorities for the health care workforce, Aiken and Salmon (1994) concluded that in terms of sheer numbers, the aggregate supply of nurses appears to be adequate for meeting national needs in the near term. However, they noted that the mix of nurses by educational background is inadequate to meet the increasing demand for nurses in leadership and advanced practice roles.

## ORIGIN, PURPOSE, AND ORGANIZATION OF THE REPORT

At the request of a consortium of federal agencies (Agency for Toxic Substances and Disease Registry, National Institute of Environmental Health Sciences, National Institute of Nursing Research, Health Resources and Services Administration, National Institute for Occupational Safety and Health, Environmental Protection Agency), and as follow-up to a planning meeting conducted by the Institute of Medicine (IOM), the IOM established the Committee on Enhancing Environmental Health in Nursing Practice to address issues related to the need for enhancing environmental health content in nursing practice. The committee was charged with the following tasks:

- assess the current status of environmental health in the practice of nursing and the need for enhanced education and research;
- provide guidance on the development of environmental health curricula for nurses;
- identify barriers to the integration of environmental health content into nursing education and the practice of nursing;
- develop implementation strategies for enhancing environmental health in nursing education, practice and research, including methods and resources for faculty development;
- describe methods for evaluating the effectiveness of an enhanced environmental health curriculum; and
- identify and describe: (a) environmental health/nursing research issues, (b) potential roles for government, industry, and academia in supporting environmental health/nursing research and practice, and (c) potential collaborative and interdisciplinary activities and research initiatives that might be undertaken in addressing environmental health/nursing issues.

The report offers some starting points for considering what kinds of change are needed and what kinds of change are possible with respect to enhancing the environmental health content in nursing practice, and should be of interest to nurse educators, practicing nurses, and other professionals who interact with nurses to promote the health of the public. First, it provides factual information about the present status of the environmental health content in nursing practice, education, and research. Second, it clarifies some of the complex reasons for the present neglect of this subject area in professional nursing. Third, it proposes some strategies for enhancing the training, skills, and roles of nurses so that they are better able to make the connection between environment and health and more empowered to help the patients and populations affected by environmental health hazards.

Following this introduction, Chapter 2 outlines some of the environmental health hazards of concern. The subsequent three chapters examine, in turn, the complexities of enhancing environmental health content in nursing practice, education, and research. The analysis and discussion in each chapter concludes with some recommendations for change that would improve nursing by enhancing the emphasis on environmental health. Eight appendixes are included at the end of the report: (A) *The Nurse's Role in Safeguarding the Human Environment* (ICN, 1986); (B) Environmental Hazards for the Nurse as a Worker; (C) *Environmental Health Curricula* (Lipscomb, 1994a); (D) Environmental Health Resources: Agencies, Organizations, Services, and General References; (E) Focus Group Summary and Lists of Focus Group Participants; (F) Nursing Advocacy at the Policy Level: Strategies and Resources; (G) Taking an Environmental Health History; (H) Acknowledgments; and (I) Committee and Staff Biographies.

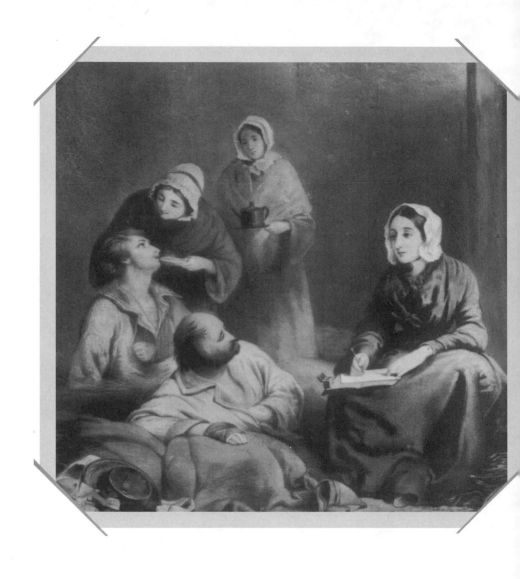

*"I was sick and ye visited me."*
*Florence Nightingale at Therafia Hospital,*
*near Constantinople, Turkey.*

*Photogravure (1855).*
*Property of Duke University Medical Center Library,*
*History of Medicine Collections, Durham, NC.*

# 2

# Overview of Environmental
# Health Hazards

*The most difficult challenges for environmental health today come not from what is known about the harmful effects of microbial agents; rather they come from what is not known about the toxic and ecologic effects of the use of fossil fuels and synthetic chemicals in modern society.*

—DHHS, 1990, p. 312

Environmental health hazards are ubiquitous, affecting all aspects of life and all areas of nursing practice. As noted by the National Research Council in 1984, more than 65,000 new chemical compounds have been introduced into the environment since 1950, and new chemical compounds enter commerce each year. The post-World War II era brought major technological advances to society, accompanied by the release of an unprecedented amount of synthetic chemicals onto U.S. markets. It is presently estimated that there are 72,000 chemicals currently used in commerce (excluding food additives, drugs, cosmetics, and pesticides), the majority of which have had limited testing for their effects on human health and the environment (INFORM, 1995). Even less is known about simultaneous exposures to a number of different chemicals, which is how most human contact with chemicals occurs.

As early as 1979, the Surgeon General's Report on Health Promotion and Disease Prevention noted, "There is virtually no major chronic disease to which environmental factors do not contribute, either directly or indirectly" (DHHS, 1979, p. 105). Nevertheless, it is impossible to accurately quantify the burden of morbidity and mortality related to environmental exposures for several reasons: poor compliance with reporting requirements for occupational illness, long latency periods between initial exposure and resulting disease, the inability of health care providers to recognize environmental etiologies of diseases, and the absence of national reporting systems for environmentally related illnesses. The extent of the problem is further obscured by the multifactorial etiology of many environmentally related diseases (e.g., lung cancer caused by exposure to asbestos is more likely to occur among people who smoke tobacco). Nevertheless, the link between adverse health effects and exposure to environmental hazards has been well established, and much can be done to prevent or minimize environmentally related illnesses.

While scientific understanding of the potential adverse health effects of most chemical compounds on humans is incomplete, reports concerning the adverse health affects associated with chemical exposures in other species are frequent. People's concerns about the impact of environmental conditions on their health are often voiced to nurses in the community and at the workplace. However, many nurses do not have the knowledge needed to identify environmental factors that may contribute to illness and injury among the populations they serve.

Environmental hazards may be encountered at home, work, or in the community via several *pathways*: contaminated air, soil, water, and food (see Figure 2.1). *Routes of exposure* include: inhalation, such as, of dust or fumes; ingestion, such as, of pesticide residues on fruits and vegetables; and dermal absorption, such as, of ultraviolet-B radiation from the sun or direct skin contact with caustic household cleansers.

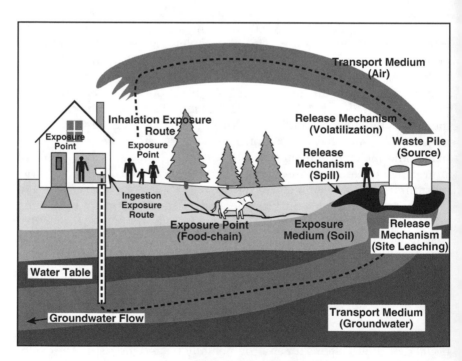

**FIGURE** 2.1 Exposure pathways. SOURCE: ATSDR, 1992.

This chapter provides an overview of environmental hazards to human health in the home, workplace, community, and globally. It is only an overview, and does not include all environmental hazards or all environmentally related illnesses, nor does it detail all of the hazards to, or specific vulnerabilities of, various subpopulations. It does, however, establish a basis for the need to examine the role of nurses in addressing environmental health issues, particularly for readers who are new to the field of environmental health. Subsequent chapters will link the problems described in this chapter to implications for changes in nursing practice, education, and research to allow for more effective interventions in matters of environmental health.

## CLASSIFYING HAZARDS

Although a number of systems are used to characterize environmental hazards, most commonly they are classified as either chemical, physical, mechanical, or psychosocial hazards. Table 2.1 presents this classification scheme, along with examples of hazards that fall into each category. Stevens and Hall (1993) have compiled a list of environmental health problems that are categorized by a variety of broad public health issues (Table 2.2), which is also included to illustrate the range of specific environmental problems that may adversely affect human health.

## AIR, SOIL, AND WATER

According to EPA, more than 40 million people live within 4 miles of a Superfund[1] site, and approximately 4 million reside within 1 mile of a site (NRC, 1991). Those people who live near Superfund sites may be at risk for exposure to hazardous substances in contaminated drinking water, contaminated soil in such areas as playgrounds and gardens, or through the siting of homes on contaminated property with the possibility of exposure to toxic substances via numerous routes and pathways.

Safe drinking water is a significant environmental health concern: currently 25 percent of community water systems provide drinking water that does not meet EPA safety standards for biological and chemical contaminants (DHHS, 1990). Contaminated drinking water can be a result of point-source pollutants such as Superfund sites or non-point sources such

---

[1]Superfund sites are hazardous waste sites designated by the U.S. Environmental Protection Agency (EPA) as a threat to human health. These areas may include leaking underground storage tanks or inactive hazardous waste sites such as municipal dumps and contaminated factories or mines and mills (Chiras, 1994).

**TABLE 2.1** Common Classes of Environmental Health Hazards, with Examples

| Chemical | Physical | Biological | Mechanical[a] | Psychosocial |
|----------|----------|------------|---------------|--------------|
| Lead | Noise | Bacteria | Vibration | Violence |
| Carbon monoxide | Ionizing radiation | Parasites | Repetitive motion | Stress |
| Benzene | Electromagnetic fields | Viruses | Lifting | High-demand/ Low-control occupations |
| Vinyl chloride | Temperature extremes | Vectors | | |

[a]This category is sometimes included in the class of physical hazards.

as runoff of agricultural fertilizers and pesticides into waterways that supply drinking water.

The environmental exposure limits designed to protect against contaminants may be in the form of regulatory standards (e.g., maximum contaminant levels (MCLs) for drinking water), action standards (e.g., soil lead levels exceeding 500 ppm), or risk-based standards (e.g., a $10^{-4}$ or $10^{-6}$ excess cancer risk). Environmental standards are often based on retrospective studies of worker exposure (a natural experimental model) or on laboratory studies using animals. A large degree of uncertainty exists when extrapolating from safe levels of exposure for workers based on an 8 hour period within a work site to ambient levels of residential exposure that may occur 24 hours a day outside the worksite (and away from safety systems such as exhaust ventilation). An even greater level of uncertainty and complexity results when studies of small laboratory animals exposed to large quantities of a single substance over a brief period of time are used as the basis for projecting health risk to humans, who are typically exposed to small quantities of multiple substances over extended periods of time.

Air pollution—both indoor and outdoor—raises another set of environmental hazards. Over 50 percent of the U.S. population lives in areas where the outdoor air did not meet EPA standards for contaminants (e.g., ozone, nitrogen dioxide, sulfur dioxide, particulates, and lead) at some time during the previous 12 months (DHHS, 1990). Most Americans spend the majority of their time indoors, either at home, school, or the workplace, where most of the exposure to foreign proteins via inhalation

**TABLE 2.2** Examples of Environmental Health Hazards

| Area | Problems |
| --- | --- |
| Living problems | • Environmental tobacco smoke<br>• Noise exposure<br>• Urban crowding<br>• Residential lead-based paint |
| Work hazards | • Toxic substances<br>• Machine-operating hazards<br>• Repetitive motion injuries<br>• Carcinogenic work exposures |
| Atmospheric quality | • Greenhouse gases and global warming<br>• Depletion of the ozone layer<br>• Aerial spraying of herbicides and pesticides<br>• Acid rain |
| Water quality | • Contamination by human waste<br>• Oil and chemical spills in waterways<br>• Pesticide/herbicide contamination of groundwater and runoff to local waterways<br>• Aquifer contamination by industrial pollutants<br>• Toxic contamination of fish and seafood |
| Housing | • Rodent and insect infestations<br>• Particulates from woodburning stoves<br>• Houses and buildings with poor ventilation systems—sick building syndrome<br>• Off-gases from carpets and plastics used in home construction |
| Food quality | • Bacterial contaminants<br>• Pesticide residues on fruits and vegetables<br>• Disruption of food chain by pollutants<br>• Chemical food additives<br>• Hormone supplements and antibiotic residues in animal food products |
| Waste control | • Use of nonbiodegradable products<br>• Contamination of air, soil, and waters due to poorly designed solid waste dumps and inadequate sewage systems<br>• Transport and storage of hazardous waste<br>• Illegal dumping of industrial waste<br>• Abandoned hazardous waste sites (including Superfund sites) |

continued on next page

**TABLE 2.2** Continued

| Area | Problems |
| --- | --- |
| Radiation | • Nuclear facility emissions<br>• Radioactive nuclear waste<br>• Radon gas seepage in homes and schools<br>• Nuclear testing<br>• Excessive exposure to X-rays<br>• Ultraviolet radiation (UVB) due to global depletion of stratospheric ozone |
| Violence | • Proliferation of handguns<br>• Pervasive images of violence in the media<br>• Violent acts against women and children<br>• Excessive incidents of violence in workplaces, schools, and community settings |

SOURCE: Adapted from Stevens and Hall, 1993.

occurs. A large proportion of asthmatics are allergic to indoor allergens, including foreign proteins, and exposure to these allergens can be reduced or minimized through various measures. According to the IOM, improved public and professional education are essential for the prevention and control of indoor allergic disease. Nursing education should emphasize the importance of recognition and proper management of these diseases (IOM, 1993). Paralleling increased pollution of both indoor and outdoor air, the incidence of childhood asthma has risen sharply in the last 2–3 decades. For some age groups (e.g., girls aged 5–14 years) the incidence has doubled or tripled (Yunginger, 1992). In addition, adverse health effects associated with indoor and outdoor air pollution disproportionately affect some populations; asthma mortality rates among African Americans are 3–5 times greater than among Caucasians (IOM, 1993).

Pesticide residues on fruits and vegetables, and the bioaccumulation of chemicals in fish and seafood are additional concerns: it is estimated that 25 percent of all rivers, lakes, and streams in the United States cannot support "beneficial uses," including fishing and swimming, due to widespread pollution (DHHS, 1990). Contaminants with the potential to adversely affect human health include polychlorinated biphenyls (PCBs) and mercury. Disadvantaged populations who consume larger quantities of contaminated fish caught in local waters experience a greater burden of exposure than members of other socioeconomic groups. Nurses working in community and public health settings could assist in educating the public about the hazards (or safety) of diets that consist of fish and seafood taken from local waterways and by explaining appropriate measures for rinsing pesticide residues from fruits and vegetables.

## THE WORKPLACE ENVIRONMENT

The workplace is an important setting to consider when studying environmentally related illness; environmental hazards and exposures can be substantial in occupational settings. At present, workplace injuries and fatalities are the most well-documented indices of adverse effects of the environment on health. More than 2.25 million work-related illnesses and injuries were reported to the U.S. Department of Labor in 1993 (BLS, April 26, 1995). Three primary occupations with at least 100,000 cases involving work absences[2]—truck drivers, nonconstruction laborers (except farm), and nursing aides and orderlies—had larger shares of the injury and illness case total for 1993 than their share of the total workforce (BLS, May 15, 1995). Sprains and strains were by far the leading **type** of injury, and the parts of the body most often affected were the back, shoulder, and other areas of the upper trunk. The three most common injuries or illnesses in terms of number of lost work days were carpal tunnel syndrome (median = 30 lost days), amputation (median = 22 lost days), and fractures (median = 20 lost days). Men accounted for a larger share (two-thirds) of the survey-wide total absences due to injuries and illnesses than their share (55 percent) of total employment. Women injured on the job accounted for a larger share of repetitive motion disorders (64 percent) and injuries from violent acts (57 percent) than their share of total employment (45 percent).

The costs to employers and society of these injuries are high and can be measured in lost work days: 20 percent of injured people were absent from work for 31 days or more. There were 117,000 absences in 1993 from work due to work-related *illnesses*, including carpal tunnel syndrome and long-term latent diseases, such as skin cancer following exposure to arsenic or ionizing radiation. The incidence of occupational diseases is believed to be understated in the survey because of: (1) the difficulty in relating these illnesses to the workplace, and (2) the failure of health care providers to recognize and report such conditions as being work related (BLS, April 26, 1995).

A total of 6,271 fatal work injuries were reported to the BLS in 1993—highway traffic incidents were the most common cause of death (20 per-

---

[2]An "absence" is defined as one or more work days lost due to a single episode of occupational injury or illness. Thus, five lost work days due to a sprained ankle equals one absence.

cent), followed by homicide (17 percent). Among women in the work-place, homicide was the most frequent cause of death, accounting for 39 percent of their 481 fatal injuries (BLS, May 15, 1995). Gunshot wounds were the cause of death in 82 percent of all workplace homicides. Vio-lence, and the psychosocial conditions that surround violent behavior, is an environmental hazard of epidemic proportions in the home, commu-nity, as well as in the workplace. Nurses encounter the results of violence in a number of work settings; opportunities for prevention are dependent upon recognition of factors that contribute to violence (e.g., stress, inad-equate coping skills, and poor worker–management relationships). Be-cause they frequently conduct their practice in the home, community, and workplace, nurses are often able to directly recognize these factors first-hand.

Nurses are by far the largest group of health professionals providing care in occupational settings (DHHS, 1988). This proximity to the work-place can enable nurses to identify and initiate measures to remediate workplace health hazards if they are adequately educated to do so. Nurses must also recognize a professional obligation to advise employees and employers of real or potential hazards, and where necessary, initiate steps to control or eliminate hazardous conditions.

## THE GLOBAL ENVIRONMENT

In addition to exposures at home, in the workplace, and in the com-munity, global environmental conditions may also adversely affect hu-man health. Global warming trends over the last century may have nu-merous untoward health effects should they continue. For example, it is estimated that mortality during prolonged heat waves may increase 30 percen–50 percent in U.S. cities if warming trends continue (Kilbourne, 1990). Increases in temperature may adversely affect people with a num-ber of major categories of disease, particularly cardiovascular, cerebrovas-cular, and respiratory diseases (Haines, 1993). Cardiovascular mortality associated with heat waves of 41° C may be due to a rise in heart rate of about 30 beats per minute and a fall in blood pressure that has been demonstrated under such conditions (Keatinge et al., 1986). Morbidity and mortality due to infectious diseases may also increase, as some or-ganisms now restricted to tropical areas could invade densely populated areas further north as the planet warms (Chiras, 1994).

Depletion of stratospheric ozone by the release of chlorofluorocar-bons (CFCs), which has occurred over the Arctic as well as the Antarctic, leaves large populations worldwide at risk for adverse health effects from overexposure to ultraviolet radiation. On a seasonal basis, ozone-de-pleted vortices (large air streams) break into clumps and flow from the

Antarctic over highly populated areas of Australia, New Zealand, South America, and Africa; from the Arctic, ozone-depleted air flows southward over North America and Europe. During these periods, which last for several months, ultraviolet radiation can increase by as much as 20 percent. Exposure to ultraviolet radiation is associated with a variety of adverse health effects (Miller, 1993). The incidence of melanomas has already increased by 83 percent in the United States during the period from 1982 through 1989, and the incidence of skin cancer will continue to increase with continued depletion of the ozone layer (CDC, 1995; Chivian et al., 1993; Longstreth, 1990). Low-intensity ultraviolet radiation (UV-B) from sunlight also alters T-lymphocyte function, thus suppressing cellular immunity and increasing susceptibility to carcinogenic and infectious agents (Daynes, 1990; Hersey et al., 1983). Studies of fishermen on the Chesapeake Bay have demonstrated an increased risk for cataracts associated with exposure to sunlight, an outcome believed to be related to oxygen free radicals generated by UV-B (Chivian et al., 1993; Hu, 1990; Jacques and Chylack, 1991; Rosenthal et al., 1988; Taylor, 1990).

A number of global environmental conditions have the potential for untoward effects on health, and further research is needed to illuminate these potential outcomes. Nurses who are knowledgeable about global environmental conditions, such as ozone depletion, can educate the public about measures to reduce or eliminate their exposure to such hazards, (e.g., by limiting direct exposure to the sun and through the use of sunglasses that limit transmission of ultraviolet radiation) and measures to limit further global changes that may have adverse effects on human health (e.g., by using public transportation or car-pooling when possible to reduce the production of greenhouse gases).

## VULNERABLE POPULATIONS

Individuals vary widely in their susceptibility to adverse health effects following exposure to toxic substances. Personal characteristics such as age, gender, weight, genetic composition, nutritional status, physiologic status (including pregnancy), preexisting disease states, behavior and lifestyle factors, and concomitant or past exposures may all affect human responses to environmental conditions. The manner in which these characteristics may enhance or decrease susceptibility to environmental hazards is in some cases fairly obvious, while in others it is less so. The relationship of age and genetic factors to one's susceptibility to adverse effects from environmental hazards are perhaps least obvious to clinicians. Table 2.3 summarizes some of the major genetic factors that may be associated with enhanced susceptibility to chemicals in the environment (Tarcher, 1992). The unique vulnerabilities of individuals at the

**TABLE 2.3** Genetic Factors and Susceptibility to Occupational and Environmental Chemicals

| Predisposing Factor | Incidence | Chemical(s) | Status of Genetic-Environmental Interaction |
|---|---|---|---|
| Glucose-6-phosphate dehydrogenase deficiency | About 12% among African-American males; very high in tropical and subtropical countries | Oxidizing chemicals | Likely |
| Sickle-cell trait | 7%–13% among African-Americans; 30% of population in parts of Africa | CO, aromatic amino compounds | No clear evidence |
| Methemoglobin reductase deficiency | About 1% of population are heterozygotes | Nitrites, aniline | Definite |
| Aryl hydrocarbon hydroxylase induction | High-induction-type Caucasians about 30% | Polycyclic aromatic hydrocarbons | Possible |
| Slow acetylator phenotype | Caucasians and African-Americans about 60%; Orientals about 10–20% | Aromatic amine-induced cancer | Possible |
| Paraoxonase variant | Caucasians about 50%, Orientals about 30%, African-Americans about 10% | Parathion | Possible |
| Acatalasia | Mainly Japan and Switzerland, reaching 1% in some areas of Japan | Hydrogen peroxide | Definite |
| Nontaster status | 30% Caucasians, 10% Chinese, 3% African-Americans | Goitrogens (thiourea, etc.) | Definite |
| $\alpha_1$-Antitrypsin deficiency | Homozygotes about one in 6,700 North American Caucasians | Respiratory irritants | Most likely |
| | | Smoking | Definite |
| Immotile cilia syndrome | About 1:40,000 in all major races | Respiratory irritants, smoking | Most likely |
| Immunologic hypersensitivity | Unknown, 2% in some occupational populations | Isocyanate | Definite |

SOURCE: Adapted from Tacher, A.B., ed. 1992. *Principles and Practice of Environmental Medicine.* New York: Plenum Publishing Co. Reprinted with permission.

two extremes of the life cycle, that is, young children and the aged, are similar in many ways due either to the immaturity or normal decline in functioning of major physiologic processes.

Although there are wide individual variations, elderly populations have progressively decreasing function of cardiac, renal, pulmonary, and immune system processes (Tarcher, 1992, p. 198). As a result of these changes—most of which have been documented in the study of drug therapies in the aged—elderly individuals may have impaired host defenses, impaired immune system function, and changes in their ability to detoxify chemicals. Changes in the stratum corneum of the skin can increase the percutaneous absorption of chemicals. Structural and functional changes that occur in the lung with advanced age, including loss of elasticity and impaired ciliary action, can result in more rapid absorption and decreased clearance of foreign substances in the lung. A decline in the metabolic clearance of certain drugs that require oxidative mechanisms for biotransformation has been noted in aged populations that may also result in a decreased ability to detoxify environmental toxins. Declines in blood flow to both liver and kidney, in part due to declining cardiac output estimated at 1 percent annually after the age of 30, may result in a decreased ability to detoxify and eliminate toxic substances from the body among aged populations. Immune system function is also impaired with aging, including a reduction in cell-mediated immunity and T lymphocytes. Finally, a change in body composition occurs with aging; there is a marked increase in adipose tissue mass with a decline in lean body mass. As a result of changes in body composition, water soluble drugs and chemicals have a smaller volume of distribution and greater serum levels, while lipid-soluble substances have an increased volume of distribution. This spectrum of physiologic changes in the aged may increase or decrease both their susceptibility to, and the magnitude of, adverse health outcomes associated with exposure to environmental hazards.

Children are also uniquely susceptible to environmental hazards. They have a higher basal metabolic rate than adults, which affects the absorption and metabolism of toxicants. Children also have a different breathing zone than adults; they are closer to the floor, where dust, dirt, and toxic heavy metals such as lead are deposited. The rapid growth and differentiation of cells in young children leaves them more susceptible to genetic alterations associated with many chemical exposures. An increased rate of cell proliferation can indirectly lead to carcinogenesis by increasing the likelihood that spontaneous mutation will occur or by decreasing the time available to repair DNA damage (NRC, 1993b). Moreover, the normal hand-to-mouth activity of toddlers increases the likelihood of exposure through ingestion of toxic substances. Because some toxicants are retained in "biologic sanctuaries" (e.g., lead in bone and polycyclic aromatic hydrocarbons in fat), they can cause low-dose chronic exposure for a much longer period of time than would be experienced by exposed adults. Nurses caring for children in any setting—inpatient pediatric units, well-child clinics, home health agencies, and prenatal health centers—need to understand these factors if they are to detect, or more importantly, prevent adverse environmental exposures in children.

It is estimated that 3–4 million U.S. children have blood lead levels above the defined toxic level of 10 mcg/dl, a level known to cause irreversible deficits in attention and IQ scores (ATSDR, 1988; CDC, 1991a; Needleman et al., 1979, 1990). Although lead was banned from household paint in 1971, almost all houses built before 1960 and 20 percent of those built between 1960 and 1974 contain leaded paint (Needleman and Landrigan, 1994). Children at greatest risk for lead poisoning are those living in poorly maintained, substandard housing (e.g., those living in poverty-level conditions). Nurses, including nurse practitioners, must be alert to the risk factors for lead poisoning in young children and aware of measures to reduce those risks. As recommended by the CDC, nurses and other health care providers need to phase-in virtually universal screening of children for blood lead levels (CDC, 1991a). Other environmental hazards in the home that are of concern to both children and adults include radon, environmental tobacco smoke (DHHS, 1986; NRC, 1986), pesticides (Environmental Studies Board, 1988; Miller, 1993; Moses, 1993; Sherman, 1988; Tarcher, 1992), carbon monoxide and airborne particulates from wood-burning stoves (American Thoracic Society, 1990; Samet et al., 1987; Tarcher, 1992), nitrogen dioxide from natural gas stoves (Samet et al., 1987; Tarcher, 1992), formaldehyde and other chemicals that are released as "off-gases" from new carpets, blown-in foam insulation, and synthetic materials covering the indoor surfaces of many mobile homes (Leikauf, 1992; Needleman and Landrigan, 1994; Sherman, 1988; Tarcher, 1992).

## ENVIRONMENTAL HEALTH PRIORITIES

Priority environmental hazards and environmentally related illnesses have been established by various public and private-sector organizations, including EPA, NIOSH, and the Agency for Toxic Substances and Disease Registry (ATSDR). A description of priority health conditions that were established by ATSDR is presented here as an example.

ATSDR is an agency of the U.S. Public Health Service responsible for investigating health effects related to hazardous wastes. ATSDR (Lybarger et al., 1993) classifies hazardous substances according to adverse health outcomes associated with a substance; their priority health conditions include:

- birth defects and reproductive disorders,
- cancer,
- immune function disorders,
- kidney and liver dysfunction,
- lung and respiratory diseases, and
- neurotoxic disorders.

ATSDR uses their priority health conditions to guide the use of resources in the evaluation of community health risks, in establishing health education programs, and in preventing or mitigating adverse health effects resulting from exposure to hazardous environmental agents. ATSDR's 10 leading priority environmental hazards are listed in Table 2.4.

## CONCLUSION

In conclusion, a large spectrum of environmental agents are potential health hazards. Some of these are common, others are not; some are apparent, others are not. All are important, however, and nurses need to be aware of them in their daily practice to improve the level of health care they provide. To this end, the remainder of the report addresses various aspects of enhancing environmental health in nursing practice, education, and research.

**TABLE 2.4** Agency for Toxic Substances and Disease Registry 1993
Priority List of Rank Ordered Top 10 Hazardous Substances

| Hazardous Agents | Sources | Exposure Pathways | Systems Affected |
|---|---|---|---|
| Lead | Storage batteries; manufacture of paint, enamel, ink, glass, rubber, ceramics, chemicals | Ingestion, inhalation | Hematologic, renal, neuromuscular, GI, CNS |
| Arsenic | Manufacture of pigments, glass, pharmaceuticals, insecticides, fungicides, rodenticides; tanning | Ingestion, inhalation | Neuromuscular, skin, GI |
| Metallic mercury | Electronics, paints, metal and textile production, chemical manufacturing, pharmaceutical production | Inhalation, percutaneous and GI absorption | Pulmonary, CNS, renal |
| Benzene | Manufacture of organic chemicals, detergents, pesticides, solvents, paint removers | Inhalation, percutaneous absorption | CNS, hematopoietic |
| Vinyl chloride | Production of polyvinyl chloride and other plastics; chlorinated compounds; used as a refrigerant | Inhalation, ingestion | Hepatic, neurologic, pulmonary |
| Cadmium | Electroplating, solder | Inhalation | Pulmonary, renal |
| Polychlorinated biphenyls | Formerly used in electrical equipment | Inhalation, ingestion | Skin, eyes, hepatic |
| Benzo(a)pyrene | Emissions from refuse burning and autos, used as laboratory reagent, found on charcoal-grilled meats and in cigarette smoke | Inhalation, ingestion, and percutaneous absorption | Pulmonary, skin, eyes (BaP is a probable human carcinogen) |

**TABLE 2.4** Continued

| Hazardous Agents | Sources | Exposure Pathways | Systems Affected |
|---|---|---|---|
| Chloroform | Aerosol propellants, fluorinated resins, produced during chlorination of water, used as a refrigerant | Inhalation, percutaneous absorption, ingestion | CNS, renal, hepatic, mucous membrane, cardiac |
| Benzo(b)-fluoranthene | Cigarette smoke | Inhalation | Pulmonary |

NOTE: CNS = central nervous system; GI = gastrointestinal.

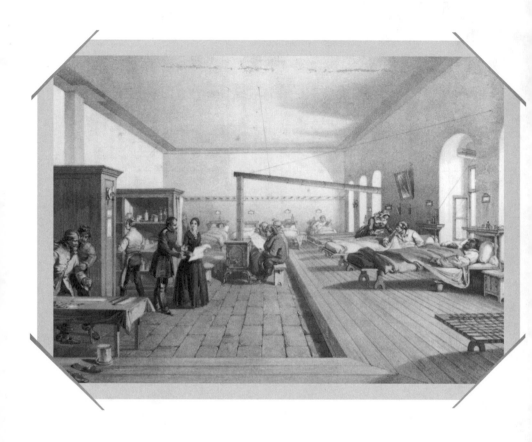

*Florence Nightingale entering one of the wards*
*of the hospital at Scutari with an officer.*

*Colored lithograph (1856).*
*Property of Duke University Medical Center Library,*
*History of Medicine Collections, Durham, NC.*

# 3

# Nursing Practice

*In watching diseases, both in private homes and in public hospitals, the thing which strikes the experienced observer most forcibly is this, that the symptoms or the sufferings generally considered to be inevitable and incident to the disease are very often not symptoms of the disease at all, but of something quite different—of the want of fresh air, or of light, or of warmth, or of quiet, or of cleanliness, or of punctuality and care in the administration of diet, of each or of all of these.*

—Florence Nightingale, 1860, p. 8

Environmental determinants of health and disease are pervasive and integral to the  assessment, diagnosis, intervention, planning, and evaluation components of nursing practice. However, environmental factors that affect health are commonly overlooked in routine patient assessments. When environmental health concerns are missed, an opportunity for prevention is lost, and public health is less well served.

Although not every illness has an environmental etiology, nearly everyone will have a health problem related to an environmental hazard for which evaluation or advice is appropriate in terms of good nursing practice. It is important in nursing practice to identify not only the hazards that contribute to a current diagnosis (e.g., exposure to lead-contaminated dust resulting in elevated blood lead levels, and outdoor ozone or indoor allergens exacerbating childhood asthma), but also those that have not yet caused illness but are amenable to intervention (e.g., friable asbestos, radon, formaldehyde gases from building materials, and carbon monoxide and nitrogen oxides from poorly ventilated furnaces). By taking a proactive approach, nurses can initiate preventive actions to abate hazards before they manifest as disease. Thus, consideration of environmental health concepts as a core nursing function will vastly strengthen nursing's contribution to disease prevention.

## NURSING PRACTICE AND RESPONSIBILITIES IN ENVIRONMENTAL HEALTH

The practice of nursing is guided by standards and definitions established by leaders of nursing in professional associations and to some extent by governmental agencies such as the Public Health Service's Bureau of Health Professions. Systematic frameworks for the practice of nursing also guide nurses in actual nursing performance. The most widely accepted framework for nursing practice currently in use is the *nursing process* of assessment, diagnosis, planning, intervention, and evaluation. A model to guide medical and nursing practice specific to environmental health concerns established by the California Public Health Foundation (CPHF, 1992) consists of three roles: investigator, educator, and advocate.

Awareness of the formal descriptions, definitions, and systems of nursing practice is useful for determining how environmental health concepts and related activities fit into nursing as it is currently practiced. A brief overview of the definitions and systems that guide nursing practice and their application to environmental health concerns is presented in the following section to demonstrate the "fit" between nursing practice and environmental health issues. The integration of environmental health concerns into nursing's scope of practice and the profession's philosophy of health and health care also illustrate nursing's historic and continued concern about environmental influences on human health.

### Definition of Nursing Practice

The American Nurses Association (ANA) provides leadership in determining the goals, objectives, and professional practice of nursing. ANA defines nursing as ". . . a caring-based practice in which processes of diagnosis and treatment are applied to human experiences of health and illness" (ANA, 1994).

ANA describes three basic nursing activities that explicitly include issues related to the environment and health, a preventive approach to health, and concern for populations as well as individuals:

1. *Restorative* practices modify the impact of illness and disease.
2. *Supportive* practices are oriented toward modification of relationships or the environment to support health.
3. *Promotive* practices mobilize healthy patterns of living, foster personal and familial development, and support self-defined goals of individuals, families, and communities.

Thus, major concepts and activities necessary to address environmental factors that can affect the health of individuals and populations are within the scope of practice and definition of nursing set forth by the ANA.

## The Nursing Process

The nursing process, consisting of assessment, diagnosis, planning/ outcomes, intervention, and evaluation, has been described as the core and essence of nursing, central to all nursing actions. It is a deliberate, logical, and rational problem solving process whereby the practice of nursing is performed systematically. The nursing process includes continuous input from patients, their families, or communities through all phases from assessment to evaluation. Diagnoses, planning, and interventions may be altered at any stage based upon new information from the patient or any other source. As far as possible, the patient should have an active and equal role in the nursing process, constricted only by physical or emotional limitations on their ability to participate.

It is worth noting that the nursing process was developed for the care of individuals, and has since expanded to include a role in the care of families and communities. Application of the nursing process to environmental health issues may require nurses to employ various phases of the process in new ways. For example, the intervention may be recommending a change in the source of drinking water that affects a whole neighborhood or community. The process is compatible with the framework of investigator, educator, and advocate, established by the California Public Health Foundation (1992) to address nursing roles and responsibilities particular to environmental health issues. The CPHF framework augments rather than duplicates the nursing process.

During the *assessment* phase of the nursing process, data are gathered to determine a patient's state of health and to identify factors that may affect well-being. This activity includes eliciting a health history to identify previous illnesses and injuries, allergies, family health patterns, and psychosocial factors affecting health. Environmental health components of history taking can be integrated into the routine assessment of patients by including questions about prior exposure to chemical, physical, or biological hazards and about temporal relationships between the onset of symptoms and activities performed before or during the occurrence of symptoms. During an assessment, the nurse should be alert to patterns of co-morbidity among patients, family members, and communities that are indicative of environmental etiologies. Nurses also conduct assessments during visits to patients in their homes and places of work, gaining first hand information about environmental factors that may adversely affect health.

*Diagnosis* occurs with the culmination of objective and subjective data collection. In this phase of the nursing process health problems are identified and described. Depending upon their practice setting, nurses may use the diagnostic terms established by the North American Nursing Diagnosis Association (NANDA) or medical diagnostic terminology, as is often the case with APNs who are nurse practitioners. Routine consideration of environmental factors that affect health is essential in the diagnostic phase of the nursing process; without knowledge of such factors, problems may be misdiagnosed and subsequent interventions will address environmental issues haphazardly, if at all.

*Planning/outcomes* is the phase of the nursing process in which optimal outcomes are identified. A range of interventions are identified to address the health problem, and plans for implementing those interventions are developed. The ability to establish interventions that address environmentally related illnesses depends on a nurse's ability to formulate diagnoses that include consideration of environmental factors. Without attention to environmental factors, intervention plans are likely to focus on secondary- and tertiary-level activities (care and cure) rather than primary prevention strategies.

*Intervention* is the component of the nursing process in which the nurse implements activities to promote health, and prevent or alleviate illness and injury. The nurse may act as educator in this part of the nursing process, informing patients, families, workers, and communities about hazards in the environment and how to protect themselves. Effective interventions require a knowledge of resources, including texts, databases, and professional experts, and an ability to access these resources.

Intervention also includes the role of advocate. Although nurses are familiar with the concept of advocacy on behalf of individual patients, often they have not been trained in techniques of advocacy for populations or in settings other than health care facilities. Nurses need to extend the concept of advocacy to include activities on behalf of communities and other groups and in settings such as the workplace or community meetings. This extension of nursing advocacy is often essential for addressing environmentally related health issues because they are frequently intertwined with social and political factors. Interventions focusing exclusively on the individual patient are rarely effective as primary prevention methods in matters of environmental health.

*Evaluation*, the final step in the nursing process, can be conducted on numerous levels and frequently results in additional interventions. The health outcomes of an individual are one method of determining the effectiveness of nursing interventions. Another measure of effective intervention in environmentally related illness is an evaluation of hazard abatement methods. Has the hazard been contained or removed from the environment of the individual? Are others living in the area protected from exposure? Evaluation should also include an assessment of the effectiveness of interventions directed toward other populations at similar risk, for example, other family members, co-workers, and community members. Were the existence of the hazard and protective measures communicated clearly and consistently to those at risk? Was effective treatment provided to others at risk who experienced symptoms? Are measures being taken to prevent similar incidents of exposure in the future? Are the patient, work population, and community satisfied with the interventions used to identify and abate hazardous conditions related to the environment? Are those affected by the hazard satisfied with the health care that was provided, including educational interventions and medical treatment? These questions and the answers to them provide nurses and other health care providers with important information for determining the effectiveness of interventions undertaken in a particular incident and in identifying more effective measures for dealing with similar problems in the future.

Application of the nursing process to environmental health concerns requires an expansion of the tools and processes used to assess patients, reason diagnostically, and develop treatments and interventions that consider environmental factors. Responsibilities for implementing clinical services relevant to environmental health will vary according to practice settings; however, the nursing process is a useful framework for applying environmental health concepts in all settings and roles.

## Scope of Responsibilities

A nurse's role in addressing environmental health issues can be conceptualized in a variety of ways. The nursing process can be augmented or integrated with other models of practice, such as the CPHF model, which consists of three roles for the health professional: investigator, educator, and advocate (CPHF, 1992). The role of investigator supports the assessment and evaluation phases of the nursing process, while the roles of educator and advocate would be carried out as interventions. This framework incorporates a range of activities, including working with communities and on matters of public policy, that may be unfamiliar to nurses who structure their practice within the more traditional framework of the nursing process applied to individual patient care.

### Role as Investigator

Nurses may act as investigators by

• taking careful environmental health histories and looking for trends in exposure, illness, and injury;

- being alert to environmental factors that influence health;
- working with interdisciplinary teams and with agencies to determine if an environmental exposure is affecting the health of a community;
- initiating or engaging in research to identify and control environmental exposures that adversely affect human health; and
- working with public and private institutions to perform risk and hazard assessments.

In actual practice, this role may include home visits to look for peeling or chipping lead paint in the residences of young children or to identify the use of poorly vented wood stoves in the home of an asthmatic child. It may also involve entering a work site to assess conditions that affect worker health and safety, including ergonomic hazards, chemical exposures, or mechanical hazards such as poorly guarded conveyor belts. Moreover, the practice of nursing itself is uniquely hazardous. A discussion of the hazards to nurses (and other health care workers) is presented in Appendix B.

One example of a nurse as investigator is a situation that occurred in 1992 in Brownsville, Texas, a town on the Mexican border. A nurse working in the labor and delivery department of a local community hospital noticed what seemed to be an unusual number of neonates born with a relatively rare but devastating birth defect, anencephaly. The nurse subsequently reviewed all birth records for the previous year and found that the incidence of children born with this defect in her facility was significantly greater than the national rate: 30 cases per 10,000 births versus 10 cases per 10,000 births, respectively. Further investigations suggested contamination of groundwater and surface water sources with chemicals known to cause adverse health outcomes of this nature (Suro, 1992) (see Box 3.1).

Eliciting an environmental health history, another investigative activity, is one of the most important actions for enhancing the environmental health content in nursing practice, because information derived from the history is essential to all other nursing activities related to environmental health. Through the environmental history, a nurse may uncover exposures to hazardous substances that neither the patient nor the clinician had suspected as etiologic agents of existing symptoms or disease. Methods and tools for taking a complete environmental health history have been well described (Goldman and Peters, 1981; Tarcher, 1992). Sample forms for taking a comprehensive environmental health history are included in Appendix G. Three key questions to be included in all histories of adult patients are the following:

---

**Box 3.1**
**Sentinel Health Events and Disease Clustering**

Environmental health concerns often surface in a community when residents or others notice an unusual pattern of illness, for which an environmental cause is suspected. Perhaps residents notice "too many" cases of childhood leukemia in a particular neighborhood near a waste dump. Perhaps local health professionals discover a common disease such as asthma or breast cancer occurring in a community at much higher rates than would normally be expected. Perhaps several cases of a relatively rare disease are detected among individuals who work at the same plant or live on the same street. Suspicion might be triggered by even a single case of illness that breaks the usual profile for that disease, such as a cardiac arrest in a 20-year-old when such an event would normally occur at an older age. This might occur following exposure to carbon monoxide, fluorocarbons, or hydrocarbons, for example.

Such atypical patterns, whether in community populations or in individuals, are called *sentinel health events* (see Rutstein et al., 1983). When investigated, they may turn out to be coincidental, with no particular relationship to environmental factors, or there may have been misperceptions of the pattern in the first place (Schulte, 1988). However, they can also signal larger health problems related to environmental hazards, such as pesticide poisoning, heatstroke, lead and other heavy metal poisonings, or respiratory diseases triggered by poor air quality (DHHS, 1990).

Detection of a sentinel health event should lead to investigation of the subpopulation of individuals who may be at risk for similar adverse health effects. This population-based approach to the tracking of environmental health concerns has been formally recommended by the U.S. Department of Health and Human Services (DHHS). In 1990, that agency recommended the establishment of 35 state plans to define and track sentinel environmental diseases (DHHS, 1990). Such tracking systems lead to early detection of disease and primary prevention through the control of hazards before they cause illness in others. However, the plan requires the assistance of a workforce adequately educated in environmental health. To contribute to this effort, nurses must adopt an orientation that is somewhat different from that currently provided in their education, roles, and practice activities.

---

1. What are your current and past longest-held jobs? (For children and teenagers, the question can be modified to: Where do you spend your day, and what do you do there?)

2. Have you had any recent exposure to chemicals (including dusts, mists, and fumes) or radiation?

3. Have you noticed any (temporal) relationship between your current symptoms and activities at work, home, or other environments?

The investigative role of nurses may extend to their being part of a community or interdisciplinary public health assessment team. The Assessment Protocol for Excellence in Public Health (NACHO, 1991) and ATSDR's Public Health Assessment process (Lybarger et at., 1993) involve identifying risk factors and exposures that affect the health of the community. Both processes also emphasize soliciting and incorporating community health concerns as part of the assessment. Nurses skilled in interviewing, active-listening, and group processes, as well as epidemiological methods, can be invaluable team members.

## Role as Educator

Nurses have long served as patient educators; they teach patients how to get out of bed following surgery, how to change a dressing, the possible side effects of medication, and the importance of diet and exercise in maintaining health. This role can be expanded to include educating patients, families, workers, and communities about the possible adverse effects of exposure to environmental hazards and how to reduce or eliminate such exposures. This type of education is commonly referred to by public agencies and environmental health specialists as hazard or risk communication.[1] Nurses can further develop this role by providing information to create environmentally safe homes, schools, day-care settings, workplaces, and communities. As role models, nurses can conduct their practice and lives in an environmentally safe manner, that is, by limiting unnecessary exposure to chemicals or by carrying out routine duties in a manner that minimizes injury due to ergonomic hazards. Nurses can act as educators by speaking at community gatherings and becoming involved in community-level activities related to the environment and human health. They may also participate in risk or hazard communication for public health agencies.

The original focus of risk communication was on developing and delivering a message from an expert or agency to the public, in order to help the public better understand a situation and its implications for their health and well-being. This definition is widening to incorporate a two-way dialogue between regulators or managers and the public (Cutter, 1993). The interactive process of exchanging information on technical hazards and the human response, both physiological and emotional, calls for professionals who can listen, interpret, clarify, and reframe questions and information in emotionally charged and sometimes hostile situations. The basic patient education role of nurses with individuals and families

---

[1]In this report, when referring to the interaction between health professionals and individuals who are potentially affected by exposure to environmental hazards, the term *risk communication* will be used.

will need expansion to include communication with entire communities and the general public if they are to fill an essential niche in environmental health. The ability to assess the target audience, develop a message that is meaningful and understandable, choose a method or media for conveying the message, and conduct community-level conflict resolution are skills beyond the current preparation of most nurses.

The basic skills of linking individual needs with information and other resources will need to be broadened to include community linkages with environmental experts who may be outside the usual network of nursing referrals. The need to expand nursing's role in environmental health is not obvious to many nurses, for several reasons. First, no role models (faculty, supervisors) have alerted them to the potential hazards of environmental exposures. As a result, nurses are not aware that certain substances are highly hazardous to human health or that certain environmental conditions are contributing significantly, although insidiously, to the morbidity and mortality of the populations they serve. Second, nurses suspect, or are questioned by their patients about, the safety of certain conditions, but they do not know where to find accurate information about environmental hazards and measures to control them. Nurses who have attended NIOSH sponsored educational programs in occupational health can assist other nurses in learning about environmental issues by acting as guest lecturers in schools of nursing and as preceptors in the field of occupational health. Further support of this nature will enhance the ability of nurse generalists to educate their patient populations about environmental health issues.

### Role as Advocate

In theory, the human health aspects of environmental problems can be isolated and dealt within traditional medical systems. In practice, these issues usually unfold in a highly charged social and political context. Nurses and other health care providers often need to help individual patients locate and secure access to specialized services for health problems related to environmental hazards. They may also be called upon to contact individuals, agencies, and organizations outside the health care system, working on behalf of patients or communities to change hazardous conditions and prevent future health problems.

It is generally agreed that the interests of patients, workers, or community members are best served by empowering them to act as their own advocates. However, nurses' scientific knowledge and experience in speaking with scientists, physicians, and other authorities equip them to be effective advocates in some situations where individual citizens are likely to feel intimidated. This role is particularly important when advocacy involves communication with public health agencies and private industry, wherein inquiries by individual citizens sometimes meet with responses that fail to address their concerns.

Establishing the legitimacy of advocacy activities as elements of nursing practice will require concerted effort among educators and leaders in the nursing profession. Environmental health issues are highly intertwined with social and political policies; thus, in the area of environmental health, advocacy is needed at the policy level as well as on behalf of individual clients. Advocacy as one component of the nurse's role is essential if a stronger, more prevention-oriented model of nursing practice is to be established. A more in-depth discussion of the practice of advocacy by nurses is provided in Box 3.2 and Appendix F.

## Interdisciplinary Aspects of Environmental Health

Environmental hazards and their health effects rarely lend themselves to simple solutions applied from a single discipline. Effective interventions for environmentally related illness require collaborative efforts from many disciplines due to the complex nature of environmental health issues, the rapidly advancing science base in environmental health, and the need for primary prevention strategies that often must involve professionals from fields other than nursing. Such collaboration includes ongoing dialogue and fluidity of roles and responsibilities.

Nurses are accustomed to working with members of other disciplines toward a shared goal, although it is often in a multidisciplinary manner, with members of each discipline performing their activities independently and with clear role delineation. Various nursing associations and other health professions advocate a more collaborative approach to health problems that is highly interactive and more likely to be termed *interdisciplinary*. This issue is important to consider in order to most effectively address environmental health issues.

The ANA's draft Nursing Social Policy Statement notes that nursing has an "external boundary" that interacts with other professions in response to changing societal needs and the advance of scientific knowledge. The boundaries are fluid rather than firmly defined, with members of various professions cooperating in the exchange of knowledge, techniques, and ideas on how to deliver quality health care. Collaborative practice, with some overlap of function, enables members of various disciplines to interact with a shared overall mission (ANA, 1994).

The National League for Nursing (NLN) has described several aspects of the complex nature of health care: technological advances that increase access to information, the need to educate professionals to recognize patterns and engage in innovative problem solving rather than sim-

## Box 3.2
## Advocacy Practice

Interventions in environmental health problems often require nurses and other health care professionals to assume the roles of advocate, activist, and policy planner on behalf of a single patient or population of patients. Patient advocacy within the health care setting is familiar to most, if not all, nurses; for example, bringing a patient's concerns to the attention of the physician. However, advocacy that goes beyond the health care system is a new kind of activity for many nurses, who may feel ill equipped to translate research and practice issues into health policy terms.

Most nursing professionals are comfortable with the idea of case advocacy on behalf of an individual patient, even when it involves aggressive action in the interests of the patient. Where ambivalence occurs is over policy-level (class) advocacy aimed at changing environmental conditions that are detrimental to populations of patients. For some members of the profession, the latter kinds of activity will seem unprofessional, overly political, and inappropriate for nurses. Others will regard it as an expression of nursing's true mission, going back to the profession's origins as crusaders for social justice, as embodied in the practice Florence Nightingale and Lillian Wald. Nurses interested in advocacy practice will find many pressures and incentives encouraging them to define this activity around the needs of individual patients. Policy-level advocacy for structural change is not emphasized in nursing education, not fully legitimized by the field's professional associations (although it is popular among student members), and not welcomed by the majority of employers and hospital administrators. In the area of environmental health, however, nurses are likely to be drawn into a fuller range of advocacy activities whether they are prepared for these roles or not. Therefore, the issue is not whether to undertake policy advocacy, but rather how to do it in a way that is sophisticated, realistic, and constructive. Anxiety about advocacy roles can be lessened considerably by building familiarity with a wider range of advocacy techniques, not all of which are necessarily adversarial.

There are many ways to conceptualize and practice advocacy in health and human services, and there are many heated debates about what true advocacy means. Different starting premises are possible. For example, who determines what is needed: the professional or those directly affected? Should professionals acting as advocates aim simply to solve the current problem, or should they, in addition, try to empower patients and communities to solve similar problems for themselves in the future? Is public conflict something always to be avoided in advocacy efforts, or is it sometimes useful? In thinking about such questions, nurses can draw on literature from other professional fields with advocacy dimensions such as social work, city planning, education, public health, law, and mediation. Based on a review of advocacy literature, Appendix F presents some useful conceptual frameworks for understanding different forms of advocacy and different advocacy strategies.

Advocacy that goes beyond helping an individual patient and enters the realm of health policy is not yet acceptable and expected practice for all nurses. To prepare the profession for a broader range of advocacy activities, nursing curriculum and continuing education programs may come to include content on lobbying, use of media, mediation, expert testimony, community organizing, and the like. In the meantime, whether with institutional support or on their own, nurses who are stretching the definitional boundaries of advocacy practice will need to build skills that were likely not part of their basic nursing education. Appendix F lists some of the self-training and support resources available for health and human services professionals interested in advocacy practice at the policy level.

ply mastering didactic content, and an increasingly broad and integrated knowledge base that is not discipline specific (NLN, 1992). These issues are particularly relevant to environmental health, a field that requires (1) an ability to access information that is current and comprehensive, (2) the ability to recognize patterns of disease, and (3) engagement in interdisciplinary actions to gain expertise from disciplines such as physics, sociology, political science, history, and ecology as well as various health disciplines.

A great deal of emphasis has recently been placed on the idea of collaboration as a component of the interdisciplinary approach:

> The ability to co-labor (collaborate) is clearly vital when the plethora of health professionals and their increasing specialization and role differentiation combine with the complexity of patient care demands to make interdependency among professionals essential (AACN, 1995).

Others have written in the same vein, stressing the urgent need for interdisciplinary training in the health professions (IOM, 1988) and collaborative practice between nurses and physicians (Fagin and Lynaugh, 1992). Unfortunately, despite the clear mandate for interdisciplinary practice, many barriers to such arrangements exist; these include restrictive licensure and practice laws and inadequate interdisciplinary education (AACN, 1995; Safriet, 1994).

Individuals practicing in public health and occupational health and their professional associations support interdisciplinary models of practice. Professions involved in addressing environmental health concerns include, but are not limited to, specialists in industrial hygiene, toxicology, safety, ergonomics, engineering, hydrogeology, medicine, and occupational health. Nurses must know the types of knowledge, functions, and practice that constitute these disciplines, and of equal importance, other health professionals must be aware of the knowledge base, functions, and practice of nurses.

Nursing offers a unique and invaluable perspective on environmentally related health issues. However, to incorporate environmental health concerns into their practice, nurses will need to function as members of interdisciplinary teams. To accomplish this, (1) training of health professionals must put greater emphasis on developing skills for interprofessional collaboration, negotiation, critical thinking, and mutual problem solving; (2) there must be opportunities for interdisciplinary interaction throughout professional education and clinical practice; and (3) existing barriers to interdisciplinary collaboration and practice must be removed.

# FACTORS THAT INFLUENCE NURSING PRACTICE

## Professional Associations

Professional associations play a significant role in influencing nursing practice so that it keeps pace with society's health care needs. They identify and address practice issues and lead the nursing community with respect to improved, expanded, and advanced practice and education. Professional associations also inform the general public about the scientific discipline of nursing and influence external bodies (e.g., governmental agencies, private foundations) in garnering support for nursing education and research.

Many professional associations are involved in additional activities, such as (1) creating standards of care to delineate the scope of practice and professional accountability, frameworks for measuring patient outcomes, and parameters for practice evaluation; (2) developing codes of ethics to guide ethical decision making and the delivery of ethically centered care; (3) supporting education and research activities (e.g., journals, continuing education programs, certification, and grants) to improve and foster nursing knowledge and contribute to professional development; and (4) supporting a governmental affairs program to influence regulatory and policy initiatives.

Professional societies can provide relevant educational opportunities and help identify mechanisms for increasing the level of integration of environmental health concepts into practice. Several national and international organizations including the ANA, the International Council of Nurses (ICN), the American Association of Occupational Health Nurses, and the International Commission on Occupational Health (ICOH) play key roles in practice, education, and research relevant to environmental and occupational health and can serve as models for other associations. The American Public Health Association, an interdisciplinary professional society, provides a forum for building consensus on emerging public health needs and disseminating innovative strategies to address these needs, including environmental health issues. Professional associations can have a major influence on the integration of environmental health concepts into general and specialty nursing practice, and they must be considered in strategies for altering nursing practice to include environmental health issues.

## Ethical Dilemmas

Environmental and occupational health issues are fraught with potential ethical conflicts. Nurses may find themselves in situations where they wish to advocate for clients or communities who are at risk for adverse environmental exposures, but the nurses fear adverse career repercussions if they do so. For example, an occupational health nurse may place her own job in jeopardy by advocating for a costly change in the workplace that would create a safer environment for workers. Nurses may encounter ethical problems related to resistance from political and community forces of many types. The very clients whose health is at risk may deny or conceal the hazard because they fear loss of their own jobs or a decline in housing values if the hazard becomes public knowledge. For example, migrant workers and farmers may be unwilling to jeopardize their income for issues of health and safety; likewise, residential and commercial development may be deemed more important to community leaders than the resulting noise, air, and water pollution.

Concern about the confidentiality of health information obtained from employees is significant, especially when occupational health nurses are threatened by managers with job termination if they do not relinquish specific health and medical information about a worker. Although companies have a right to know whether their employees are physically and mentally capable of performing a job, employees also have the right to keep specific information about their health or medical diagnoses private. This situation often creates conflicting loyalties for nurses. In such cases, nurses must be guided by professional codes of ethics, both general and specific to their area of practice.

All individuals have the right to know about actual or potential health exposures in order to make informed decisions about the protection of their own health and that of their families and future offspring. For example, if a toxic spill occurs in a community or workers are exposed to chemical toxicants, the health professional has an ethical obligation to inform all parties of the potential consequences of the exposure. In some situations, community leaders and company executives assume a paternalistic posture, believing that they know what is best in terms of information disclosure. This attitude may place certain populations at greater risk due to lack of access to health care and potential harm from continued exposure. For example, those living closest to a spill, those spending the most time near toxic substances during cleanup, and particularly sensitive populations such as children and pregnant women living in the area near a chemical spill may be at greater risk for adverse health effects than others in the community, and they should have full access to information about substances to which they have been potentially exposed. Nurses must be knowledgeable about potential hazards and may need to act autonomously in supplying the required information to community members, on the basis of professional, ethical responsibilities—whether they are explicit or implicit in nature.

Ethical dilemmas may also arise during the course of nursing research on environmental health problems, for example whether control groups should be identified and denied intervention for the purposes of a study. Other issues in environmental health intervention research are how best to protect confidentiality and how to achieve meaningful informed consent.

Resources for addressing ethical conflicts regarding environmentally related health issues must be integral components of educational preparation for nurses at all levels of practice.

## Credentialing

### Licensing

Individual licensure of nurses is conferred by meeting the eligibility requirements and achieving a passing score on the National Council Licensure Examination for Registered Nurses (NCLEX). Registered nurse (RN) licensure conveys authority for a nurse to practice within the scope of practice defined by a state. NCLEX does not directly measure the environmental health science content of the nursing curriculum, although test items may reflect nursing knowledge secondary to the understanding of underlying environmental factors. Because schools of nursing use data on the passing rate for NCLEX as an educational outcome indicator, the influence of NCLEX items and the content of this examination on curricular decisions for nursing education cannot be underestimated (see Chapter 4).

### Certification

Unlike licensure, certification is a voluntary process in which an RN seeks an additional credential in a distinct practice area. In the future, recognition as an advanced practice nurse may require both certification and licensure.

Three certifying bodies, the American Nurses Credentialing Center (ANCC), the American Board for Occupational Health Nurses, Inc. (ABOHN), and the National Board for Certification of School Nurses, Inc. (NBCSN), were surveyed and asked to describe the nature of certification for environmental health nursing. Three questions were asked: (1) Is a certification examination in environmental health sponsored by the organization? (2) Identify by test content outlines and key words those certification examinations that have environmental health concepts among the test items. (3) What data, if any, does the organization have on the need for or interest in a certification examination in environmental health?

Bowers (1994), in responding for the ANCC, stated that environmental health nursing does not have a specific certification examination. Among the 24 certification areas where examinations do exist, a review of test content found that one or more concepts of environmental health nursing could be inferred in 21 of the examinations. These were typified by "lead poisoning, safety, poisoning and air pollution."

Further analysis revealed that 19 of 24 certification areas included the word *environment* in the outline. Test content outlines of two examinations included *environmental science*: community health nurse and clinical specialist in community health nursing practice. The pediatric nurse practitioner examination content outline dedicated a section to environmental issues, and the general nursing practice test content outline noted the influence of "environmental and occupational factors" in consideration of health promotion, disease prevention, and control.

A key word search of environmental health and its derivatives (e.g., air pollution, sanitation, and safety) located the presence of at least one key word in 15 of 24 banks of items for specific examinations. Bowers reports that ANCC has not gathered data to substantiate or refute the need for a certification program in environmental health nursing and has no current plan to offer such an examination (Bowers, 1994).

The ABOHN certification exam has integrated environmental health concepts into the certifying examination. Six content domains make up the examination blueprint, one of which is labeled "health and environment relationships." This area focuses on environmental exposure in the workplace and the application of the nursing process to the health status of workers. ABOHN has not compiled data to substantiate the need for developing a certification examination in environmental health separate from an examination in occupational health.

The NBCSN includes questions on its certifying exam related to environment and human health. These questions are found under the topic areas of health promotion/disease prevention, health problems, nursing management, and emergency care.

Currently, certification in environmental health nursing does not exist for the generalist nor for those in advanced practice, although several certifying organizations report that environmental health concepts are present to some degree. Based on this survey of certifying organizations, current credentialing systems do not include the specificity and breadth of environmental health content necessary to ensure its inclusion in basic generalist practice.

## Changes in Health Care Delivery

Health care delivery is undergoing rapid change, with a pervasive trend toward institutional consolidation and emphasis on cost cutting.

The ANA (1994) has expressed concern about a number of events that are occurring with ever-increasing frequency:

- adoption of new models of care delivery without sufficient testing, including changes in workforce patterns that may cause a decline in patient safety and quality of care;
- downsizing, layoffs, and other cost containment measures, with substitution of less highly skilled personnel for RNs; and
- lack of education and redeployment strategies to ensure a supply of appropriately prepared RNs for the demands of the future.

Along with these trends, health services research has documented a statistically significant relationship between the level and mix of nursing staff in hospitals and patient outcomes (Prescott, 1993). Specifically, as the number of nurses and the percentage of RNs on staff increases, risk-adjusted hospital mortality rates decline, as does length of inpatient stay.

The ANA is concerned about the possibility of declining patient safety and adverse health outcomes, as well as the increasing stress (physical and psychological) on nurses that is likely to increase work-related injuries as a consequence of downsizing and lowered skill requirements of the patient care workforce. As noted by Redman (1994), current changes in workforce patterns at healthcare facilities are resulting in fragmentation of nursing care, with fewer opportunities for one-to-one contact of nurses with patients. The replacement of RNs with unlicensed assistant personnel (UAPs) further distances RNs from direct contact with patients. According to the ANA, almost half of the state nursing associations deem the new mix or proportions of RNs and UAPs as unsafe. To paraphrase Redman, it may be possible to get knowledge of environmental concepts into the nurse, but because of declining direct patient contact by RNs, it cannot be assumed that such environmental health concepts will be integrated into nursing practice (Redman, 1994).

Under such circumstances, the call for adding more environmental health content to nursing practice may ring very hollow to some. However, the committee is not recommending something new, but rather a return to earlier, broader views of the nursing profession that include environmental concerns. Enhancing environmental health content in nursing practice will involve an elaboration of existing skills and perspectives, such as including environmental factors in history taking and seeking methods of primary prevention to eliminate illness and injury.

## Funding for Public Health

Recent efforts toward health care reform on both federal and state levels focus attention on improving access to care for the sick through adequate insurance coverage.  Tied closely to these efforts is the concern for controlling health care costs.  Nursing leadership has firmly supported such reforms.  Not incidental to proposals by nursing leaders is the call for increasing the supply and inclusion of advanced practice nurses (e.g., nurse practitioners, clinical specialists, and certified nurse midwives) in community-based systems of primary care.  Compelling data have been compiled that demonstrate the potential to increase accessibility of care and decrease cost, without a loss of quality of care (Boex et al., 1993).

Struggling for attention in the current health care reform debates, which focus largely on care for the sick, is the message from those in public health settings that it requires more than seeing a doctor for people to stay healthy.  The public health community (e.g., state and federal governmental agencies; professional associations; and the Office of the Assistant Secretary for Health, U.S. Department of Health and Human Services [DHHS]) has been a persistent voice for a broader perspective of health care that encompasses preventive strategies as well as traditional care and cure models.

*Public Health in America* (PHS, 1994) describes the core functions of public health as follows:

- prevents epidemics and the spread of disease,
- protects against environmental hazards,
- prevents injuries,
- promotes and encourages healthy behaviors,
- responds to disasters and assists communities in recovery, and
- assures the quality and accessibility of health services.

To fulfill these core functions, public health advocates, including environmental health professionals, appeal for funding that is distinct from reimbursement of sick care services.  Strategies include a set-aside in the health care budget or a separate, reliable appropriation to carry out governmental responsibility to protect the health of populations.

Nurses, dispersed throughout the health care system, have potential for demonstrating that competent health care can be accessible, affordable, and acceptable to the public.  The heritage of nursing services designed to strengthen the populations they serve, the principles of social justice, and nursing's broad definition of health are assets for nurses who are willing to take up new and expanded practice roles that include environmental health.  Nurses' ability to see the interconnectedness of environmental influences with opportunities for preventing health problems and controlling overall system costs can be invaluable.

## CASE STUDY

The following case study (Box 3.3) illustrates the manner in which an environmentally related illness may be encountered in day-to-day practice, along with a discussion of the actions taken by various practitioners. Its purpose is to provide an initial understanding of the responsibilities a nurse or nurses must undertake to resolve environmentally-related health problems, working in interdisciplinary teams with an ultimate goal of primary prevention. It is also an example of what can happen when environmental health issues are not addressed in a timely manner.

*Responsibilities of Nurses*

Whatever their practice roles and settings nurses must be prepared to recognize the early signs and symptoms of illness that are the result of exposure to environmental hazards. In addition, practicing nurses must consider their professional responsibilities in this arena as they are applied through the nursing process. In many instances, nurses already have the tools required to assess and assist individuals, families, and communities in primary, secondary, and tertiary prevention of environmentally-related illness. Specific areas of knowledge that may be required include how to elicit an environmental health history, how to

---

**Box 3.3**
**Illustrative Case Study**

A female infant born weighing 7 pounds, 9 ounces, appeared healthy during her first month at home. However, she became ill at 3 weeks of age and developed diarrhea and vomiting after feeding. At 6 weeks of age she was hospitalized for treatment of vomiting, failure to thrive, and dehydration. She weighed 6 pounds, 10 ounces, and had no other signs of infection. The infant was rehydrated and returned to her home the following day. After 6 days at home, she was readmitted with recurrence of symptoms and a diagnosis of failure to thrive. Her blood hemoglobin level was normal; however, her methemoglobin level was 21.4 percent (normal level, 0 percent–3 percent). She was diagnosed with methemoglobinemia and treated with oral fluids and oxygen, and within 24 hours her methemoglobin level dropped to 11.1 percent. The family began using bottled water to dilute the formula, and symptoms did not recur. The family's home was situated on a river bank near 100 acres of corn and alfalfa. Water was supplied by a shallow, 28-foot standpoint well. Water samples collected from the well during the infant's hospitalization were analyzed and found to contain excess levels of nitrates, and water samples from the kitchen faucet were found to contain excess levels of copper. On the basis of these analyses, the health department recommended that the family use bottled water for drinking and food preparation.

conduct a community assessment, and techniques for communication of risk.

## Types of Prevention

Primary prevention focuses on the prevention of exposure and promotion of health. Secondary prevention occurs after a patient has been exposed to an environmental hazard and involves recognizing and reducing the adverse health effects resulting from the exposure. Tertiary prevention occurs after exposure to the environmental hazard has occurred and while the client continues to experience long-term health effects from the exposure. Interventions at the tertiary stage are rehabilitative and protective in nature. Figure 3.1 provides a diagrammatic description of the levels of prevention.

In this case study nurses may have interacted with the family in a variety of roles and settings. The infant was probably born in an inpatient setting and discharged to the home with her family. She may then have been seen in an outpatient setting for well-child and acute illness care as mentioned in the case study. In all of these settings nurses practicing as generalists as well as advanced practice nurses would be responsible for assessing the infant, the family, and to some extent, the community in which they live. At birth, nurses in the inpatient setting are responsible not only for the care of the infant but for planning to discharge the infant and mother to the home. The health history of this infant should have included an assessment of any known environmental risk. At this point, the nurse would plan and implement primary prevention strategies with the family to reduce or eliminate environmental health risks, for example, by teaching appropriate procedures for handling food and water to prevent gastrointestinal problems. This should include information on the possible sources and routes of contamination of food and water. The nurse should also teach the family how to recognize the signs and symptoms of illness that require early medical attention.

Following discharge from inpatient care, the infant was most likely seen for a well-child visit. The infant would be assessed by a generalist or advanced practice nurse for normal growth and development. In addition, anticipatory guidance and education for the care of the infant, including health promotion and disease prevention would be provided to the family.

Among the possible causes of the infant's signs and symptoms was exposure to an environmental hazard, either biological or chemical. When the infant first developed symptoms at three weeks of age, the nurse should have included an environmental health history and assessed the need for secondary prevention. The exposure history may have identi-

**Stage of Disease**

| | Susceptibility | Presympto-matic | Clinical Disease | Disability or Recovery |
|---|---|---|---|---|
| Tissue changes | Prepathogenesis | ←——— Pathogenesis ———→ | | Resolution or sequelae |
| Level of prevention | Primary | Secondary | ←——— Tertiary ———→ | |
| | | | Treatment and rehabilitation | |
| | | | Limitation of disability | |
| Modes of intervention | Health promotion and disease prevention | • Detection • Early diagnosis • Prompt treatment | | |

**FIGURE 3.1** Schematic representation of the natural history of disease and the related levels of prevention and modes of intervention. SOURCE: Adapted from Mausner and Kramer's *Epidemiology: An Introductory Text* (1985).

fied environmental hazards that would explain the cause of the infant's symptoms (contaminated drinking water). The nurse would then plan and implement secondary prevention strategies, focusing on protection of the infant and other family members from possible continued exposure. This includes parent education and referral to the local health department requesting further investigation of the home situation.

This infant was hospitalized a second time. The deterioration of her condition was due to the failure of primary and secondary prevention efforts that were aimed at correcting the infant's symptoms without knowing the etiology of the illness.

During the second hospitalization, nurses again had an opportunity for secondary prevention. Methemoglobin levels were obtained and exposure to an environmental hazard was strongly suspected. But what was the source? The nurse knew that private wells, especially in rural areas, may be contaminated with a variety of chemicals such as pesticides, nitrates, and bacteria. The nurse then contacted the local health department about the infant's illness, laboratory findings, and the diagnosis of methemoglobinemia. When one contaminant is identified or an illness that may result from water contamination occurs, it is important that the water be evaluated further.

The public health nurse scheduled a home visit to investigate the possible sources of water pollution. The visit was coordinated with the local health department sanitarian or water supply specialists. The nurse noted that the home sits on a river bank near 100 acres of corn and alfalfa. Because of the public health nurse's knowledge of environmental hazards and health risks, the nurse knew that fertilizers are one of the most common causes of nitrate contamination of drinking water.

During the visit, the public health nurse advised the family of the hazards and of ways to avoid further illness. Nitrates were the contaminant and the appropriate advice was to refrain from ingesting the water and to use only bottled water for drinking and food preparation. (In some rural areas domestic well-water nitrate concentrations are higher than 10 milligrams/liter measured as nitrogen in nitrate (ATSDR, 1991). Private wells should be tested for nitrate contamination annually. A survey conducted in Iowa found that more than 18% of rural domestic wells contain concentrations of nitrate above the regulatory level established by the Environmental Protection Agency (ATSDR, 1991).

*Need for Broad Knowledge of Environmental Hazards*

Chemical contamination of the environment affects all communities and underscores the need for all health care professionals to be knowledgeable about the exposures and related health outcomes. In this case study it is important to recognize that the most common environmental cause of methemoglobinemia in infants in the United States is ingestion of water or reconstituted formula contaminated with nitrates from agricultural fertilizers, organic animal waste, and septic sewer systems (ATSDR, 1991). Nurses can take a proactive role in identifying these hazards and providing the public with information on how to avoid exposure to nitrate-contaminated drinking water. Community assessment by interdisciplinary teams would include assessment of potential as well as actual hazards.

For the infant described in this case study, this episode of illness had a happy ending; nursing intervention and advocacy were successful. What about other infants in this community who may have been exposed to the same or similar environmental hazards?

Even though the use of bottled water for the infant's formula offered a short-term solution to the immediate health threat, the nurse's role did not end at this point. The nurse had a responsibility to assist the family in seeking long-term solutions, for example, digging a deeper well or gaining access to a community water supply that had been tested for nitrate contamination.

The nurse also needed to be sure that the U.S. Environmental Protection Agency was aware of the situation so that attention could be given to controlling the non-point-source pollution that threatened the safety of drinking water of the surrounding community. The nurse may have been able to facilitate testing of water from the wells of neighbors to assess the extent of the pollution and to institute preventive measures before others in the community were adversely affected by contamination of domestic well water. The nurse may have played a role in getting information to the community about: (1) the problem that had been identified, (2) the risks to the public's health, and (3) the appropriate actions citizens needed to take to protect themselves. Collaborating with colleagues in the field of environmental protection may have lead to the nurse's involvement in community initiatives to address the combined needs for farmers to have successful crops and for citizens to have safe drinking water.

Nurses can also intervene with agencies and organizations to protect other infants at risk. Collaborative efforts may include meeting nurse researchers from the local school of nursing who would develop a research plan to assess the problem through the collection and analysis of data. On the basis of this research, the nurses might have developed plans for educating the community on disease prevention and health promotion related to the primary source of the problem: well water contamination with chemicals used to fertilize crops. The illness of one infant and the actions of one nurse may have reduced the risks for all infants and all members of one community.

## NURSING COMPETENCIES IN ENVIRONMENTAL HEALTH

Nurses from a variety of practice settings can assist worried community residents and workers by bridging the gap between scientific information and public understanding of the environmental health risks. However, this will require nurses to view such roles as integral to nursing practice. The environmental health competencies for nurses in generalist practice presented in Box 3.4 were adapted by the committee from competencies set forth by the International Council of Nurses (Appendix A) and by Lipscomb, 1994a (Appendix C).

## CONCLUSION

The practice of nursing has historically included a consideration of environmental factors that may affect the health of individuals, communities, and other populations. Attention to environmental factors is explicitly included in the scope of nursing practice as defined by the ANA (1994). Nevertheless, for the last half-century, the major focus of nursing

---

**Box 3.4**
**General Environmental Health Competencies for Nurses**

I. *Basic knowledge and concepts*
   All nurses should understand the scientific principles and underpinnings of the relationship between individuals or populations, and the environment (including the work environment). This understanding includes the basic mechanisms and pathways of exposure to environmental health hazards, basic prevention and control strategies, the interdisciplinary nature of effective interventions, and the role of research.

II. *Assessment and referral*
   All nurses should be able to successfully complete an environmental health history, recognize potential environmental hazards and sentinel illnesses, and make appropriate referrals for conditions with probable environmental etiologies. An essential component of this is the ability to access and provide information to patients and communities, and to locate referral sources.

III. *Advocacy, ethics, and risk communication*
   All nurses should be able to demonstrate knowledge of the role of advocacy (case and class), ethics, and risk communication in patient care and community intervention with respect to the potential adverse effects of the environment on health.

IV. *Legislation and regulation*
   All nurses should understand the policy framework and major pieces of legislation and regulations related to environmental health.

practice has been on treatment of diseases in acute care settings, rather than on health promotion and disease prevention in primary care and community-based settings. With changes in health care delivery systems and the emergence of environmentally related illnesses, all nurses (not just specialists) must refocus their attention and acquire new skills to address these changes. The nursing process, ubiquitous to all areas of nursing practice, can be used to address environmental health issues with minor adaptations that can be drawn from the CPHF's model of a nurse as investigator, educator, and advocate.

Many factors influence changes in nursing practice, including professional associations, new and unfamiliar ethical dilemmas, credentialing requirements, funding for "public-health"-related activities, and overall changes in health care delivery. Barriers to and incentives for changing nursing practice to routinely include consideration of environmental health problems have been described in this chapter, along with recommendations and strategies to address these factors. The committee believes that these strategies, if implemented, will be successful in changing the practice of nursing, no matter the setting, in order to improve the health of the public.

Nurses are respected and trusted members of the community who often have firsthand knowledge of environmental hazards in the home, community, or workplace. Expansion of their roles as educators to include risk or hazard communication, and as advocates on behalf of communities and groups (class advocacy), in addition to individuals (case advocacy), will be fundamental for the success of interventions in environmentally related illness or injury.

## RECOMMENDATIONS

Nurses in every area of practice encounter environmentally induced illnesses, either knowingly or unknowingly. However, nurses cannot begin to address these issues until they are aware of a potential link between environmental conditions and disease. Nurses are often the only health care providers who enter the home, workplace, or communities of the populations they serve, which allows them to assess directly the existence of environmental hazards. Because of this on-site aspect of nursing practice, nurses are well positioned to detect and intervene at both the individual and community levels. Nurses also comprise the largest number of health care professionals in the United States, with a clearly defined mission of caring, advocacy, and health promotion. Together, these factors suggest that the enhancement of environmental health activities in nursing practice would significantly affect environmentally related health conditions and, in turn, improve the public's health.

## Scope of Responsibility

*Recommendation 3.1: Environmental health should be reemphasized in the scope of responsibilities for nursing practice.*

**Rationale**: Nurses in every area of practice encounter environmentally induced illnesses, either knowingly or unknowingly. Nurses can address these situations if they are aware of the potential links between environmental conditions and disease.

### Strategies for Achieving Recommendation 3.1:

1. Elicit an environmental health history during patient assessment (see Appendix G).
2. Interventions should include referrals to health agencies as well as to occupational and/or environmental specialists; education about prevention techniques; and site visits to the home, workplace, or community.
3. Licensure and certification examinations for all levels of nursing should include environmental health content.
4. Professional nursing associations should be encouraged to address environmental health through the development of policy recommendations, continuing education programs, codes of ethical conduct, and written standards of care.

## Availability and Accessibility of Resources

*Recommendation 3.2: Resources to support environmental health content in nursing practice should be identified and made available.*

**Rationale**: Environmental health issues are increasingly complex, and practicing nurses cannot be expected to be expert in all aspects of environmental health. Nurses need access to comprehensive resources for technical assistance in assessment, planning, intervention, and evaluation in the area of environmental health. Such resources may include nurse experts; professionals from other disciplines; written materials; and local, state, and federal public health and environmental protection agencies. Institutional policies that support access to and use of these resources will help nurses realize their potential in addressing environmentally related illnesses.

### Strategies for Achieving Recommendation 3.2:

1. Enhance distribution of Agency for Toxic Substance and Disease

Registry (ATSDR) and Association of Occupational and Environmental Clinics (AOEC) teaching modules to nursing faculty, students, and nurses currently in practice. Advertisements and announcements can be sent to members of nursing associations and placed in selected nursing publications.

2. Promote interdisciplinary approaches to environmental health issues in nursing practice, education, and research with funding support from private and public agencies and through recommendations from nursing professional associations, including American Association of Colleges of Nursing (AACN) and International Council of Nursing (ICN).

3. Nursing faculty, students, and practitioners should be made aware of environmental health resources in local, state, and federal public health and environmental agencies, through avenues such as state nursing associations, for example.

4. Institutional policies, including formal role definitions and staffing mix, must support nurses' access to resources and adequate opportunities for one-on-one contact between patients and nurses.

## Participation in Interdisciplinary Teams

*Recommendation 3.3: Nurses should participate as members and leaders in interdisciplinary teams that address environmental health problems.*

**Rationale:** The efficacious provision of environmental health services requires the expertise of a variety of professionals functioning as a well-coordinated team. Nurses need to know who these other professionals are, what they do, and how to work with them in an interdisciplinary team. Nurses must also be prepared to consult with other specialists in environmental health including, but not limited to, toxicologists, physicians, industrial hygienists, and epidemiologists.

### Strategies for Achieving Recommendation 3.3:

1. Develop experience with interdisciplinary teams in basic nursing education by calling on experts from various fields to teach selected content and to participate in learning activities involving case studies or problem solving.

2. Focus on the necessity of an interdisciplinary approach when teaching fundamental concepts of environmental health.

3. Provide nurses with a basic understanding of the knowledge base and practice of various interdisciplinary team members, including toxicologists, industrial hygienists, risk communicators, and hydrogeologists.

Such instruction may be done in basic RN education,[2] in advanced-degree programs, and through continuing education.

4. Facilitate interaction with other disciplines both within and external to the practice setting through clearly stated job expectations with the appropriate allocation of time and resources.

5. Participate as interdisciplinary team members in community and public health assessments.

### Educator Role: Risk Communication

*Recommendation 3.4: Communication should extend beyond counseling individual patients and families to facilitating the exchange of information on environmental hazards and community responses.*

**Rationale:** Nurses can build on existing interviewing and active-listening skills to provide an essential linkage among environmental scientists; medical and environmental epidemiologists; and individuals, neighborhoods, or community groups in communicating about risks and hazards.

### Strategies for Achieving Recommendation 3.4:

1. Provide educational content and student experiences with communities concerned about environmental exposures or potential disease clusters.

2. Involve nurses in planning for and as facilitators of meetings with community groups concerning environmental issues and public involvement with agency decision-making.

3. Develop additional knowledge and expertise in communicating appropriately with identified audiences and in developing the group facilitation skills required for advocacy practice (see Appendix F).

### Advocacy Roles

*Recommendation 3.5: The concept of advocacy in nursing should be expanded to include advocacy on behalf of groups and communities, in addition to advocacy on behalf of individual patients and their families.*

---

[2]Including associate degree, diploma, baccalaureate education and those programs whose basic nursing education is obtained at the master's level.

**Rationale**: Advocacy on behalf of communities and other groups (class advocacy) can be very different from advocacy on behalf of individual patients (case advocacy), and nurses must have some grounding in basic class advocacy skills.

### Strategies for Achieving Recommendation 3.5:

1. Nursing faculty and other nursing leaders must demonstrate that advocacy activities are within the realm of professional practice through formal education of nurses and by serving as role models.

2. Experts from other fields should be called upon to assist nurses in developing and building skills in advocacy practice (see Appendix F).

3. Educational resources and experiences should include interactions with expert practitioners from other disciplines, for example, social work.

4. Knowledge and skills basic to advocacy, such as group process, conflict resolution, and political and regulatory process, must be incorporated into nursing education and practice.

### Ethics

*Recommendation 3.6: Conduct research regarding the ethical implications of occupational and environmental health hazards and incorporate findings into curricula and practice.*

**Rationale**: Little research has addressed ethical issues related to occupational and environmental health hazards and how those issues are treated in nursing practice.

### Strategies for Achieving Recommendation 3.6:

1. Identify common problems in occupational and environmental health practice that have implications for the ethical treatment of patients and communities (e.g., confidentiality of worker health information, exposure to occupational and health hazards, and informed consent).

2. Include occupational and environmental health content related to ethical issues in nursing and public health curricula.

3. Address the ethical implications of occupational and environmental health hazards and their consequences in both public and private policy documents.

4. Include consideration of ethical principles related to occupational and environmental health in professional codes of ethical conduct.

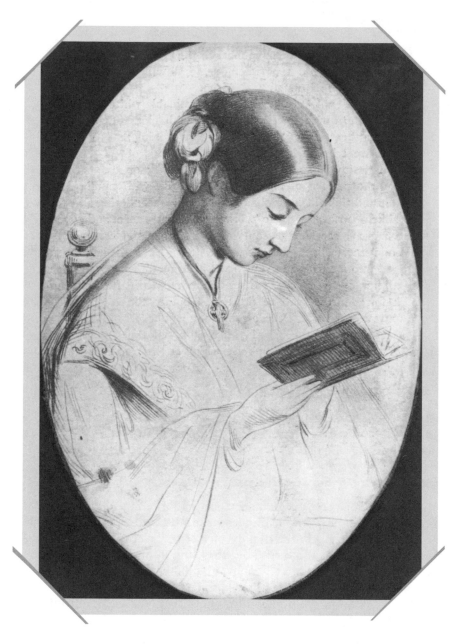

*Florence Nightingale reading.*

*Photo reproduction of an anonymous crayon drawing (1854).*
*Property of Duke University Medical Center Library,*
*History of Medicine Collections, Durham, NC.*

# 4

# Nursing Education and
# Professional Development

*The most important practical lesson that can be given to nurses is to teach them
what to observe—how to observe—what symptoms indicate improvement—
what the reverse—which are of importance—which are of none—which are the
evidence of neglect—and of what kind of neglect.*

—Florence Nightingale, 1860, p. 105

Linking the skills of professional nursing described in this quote with
the mastery of scientific knowledge of environmental health concepts
from interdisciplinary studies is essential to the reform of the educational
process for the health professions. Environmental effects on the health
and welfare of individuals, families, and communities are increasingly
complex and multifaceted. These effects require integrated knowledge of
prevention and amelioration of environmental health consequences in all
health professions education.

Of the 17 competencies of health professionals listed in *Healthy
America: Practitioners for 2005, An Agenda for Action for U.S. Health Professions Schools* (Shugars et al., 1991a), 6 directly address the demand for the
development of environmental health skills among providers: (1) understand the role of the physical environment on health; (2) respond to increased public, governmental, and third-party participation in health care;
(3) care for the community's health; (4) expand access to care and improve
the public's health; (5) emphasize prevention; and (6) promote healthy
lifestyles. These competencies illustrate the different skills, values, and
attitudes necessary to ensure improved health status outcomes in the
twenty-first century. The incorporation of environmental health concepts
and practice activities into professional education is critical for influencing health and disease outcomes worldwide.

## FACTORS AFFECTING NURSING CURRICULA

Nursing education has developed its own reforms in tandem with higher education and with other health professions education. These reforms echo the need for nursing education to reexamine the values of environmental health in policy, nursing research, education, practice, and service (AACN, 1991; ANA, 1991; NLN, 1992).

### Tradition

Although professional nursing education has traditionally included the concepts of health promotion, disease prevention, health protection, risk reduction, and population-based practice in its baccalaureate nursing degree programs, the scope and depth of such concepts and content are not consistent among programs. Commonly used nursing texts also vary in their inclusion of environmental health information. Nurses, along with physicians and pharmacists, report that the education they received regarding disease prevention was fair or poor in contrast to the excellent or good ratings of training they received regarding disease treatment or intervention (Shugars et al., 1991b).

### Trends

In *Nursing's Agenda for Health Care Reform* (ANA, 1991), three premises underlie the framework for change relative to nursing education and environmental health: (1) that primary health care plays a basic and prominent role in service delivery, (2) that a better balance exists between the prevailing orientation to illness and cure and a new commitment to wellness and care, and (3) that nursing's long-term policy agenda must consider relationships among many factors, of which environmental factors are noted. This policy document asserts that nurses who are prepared from a primary health care framework with an emphasis on prevention and environmental factors will be the providers of choice in improving the health status of the U.S. population.

Addressing nursing's need to accept the challenge of what she termed *environmental compatibility*, then-president of the American Academy of Nursing, Nola Pender, pointed out that by the year 2010, 70 percent of nurses will be practicing outside of acute-care facilities. To prepare for this shift, Pender indicates the need for curricula in schools of nursing to change. She underscores that attention in nursing education (actually, education in all health professions) should focus on high-risk environments and laments that "nursing curricula often fail to address environmental issues in-depth throughout the curriculum" (Pender, 1992, p. 201).

Nursing faculty, Pender stresses, "should determine how the concept of high risk environments may be given more attention in the curricula and which critical environmental assessment and intervention strategies are appropriate for inclusion" (Pender, 1992, p. 201).

Likewise, the American Association of Colleges of Nursing (AACN, 1991) endorses the necessity of curriculum revision to support nursing in the future. *Nursing Education's Agenda for the 21st Century* is not unlike the tenets called forth from the Pew Commission: broad content areas that are relevant to the development of healthy lifestyles and future health care solutions must be assembled. These content areas include health promotion and maintenance related to specific environmentally induced diseases (cancers, accidents and injuries, and trauma), as well as a particular emphasis on environmental and occupational health.

The traditional approach to basic nursing education represented by all three avenues— associate degree, diploma, and baccalaureate nursing programs—has been to emphasize curriculum for micro-level, individual situations rather than the macro-level of intervention. Recognizing that this individual focus will not suffice for the needs of the twenty-first century, the National League for Nursing (NLN) emphasized that "preparing all graduates of nursing education for community-based care, therefore becomes the responsibility of all programs and all faculty— perhaps in varying degrees, but a commonly shared responsibility" (NLN, 1992, p. 12).

The Association of Community Health Nursing Educators (ACHNE) published two documents describing the essentials of baccalaureate- and master's-level education for entry into community health nursing practice (ACHNE, 1992) and advanced practice nursing (ACHNE, 1991). Both documents build on reports from the American Nurses Association (ANA 1980, 1986), the World Health Organization (WHO, 1978), the American Association of Colleges of Nursing (AACN, 1986), the American Public Health Association (APHA, 1980), the U.S. Department of Health and Human Services (DHHS, 1988), and Jones et al. (1987). The community health content in the baccalaureate degree program specifies the inclusion of introductory environmental health and environmental hazards as essential to support the nurse generalist practice in the community (ACHNE, 1992). The content of the master's program to prepare advanced practice nurses in community and public health nursing specifies environmental health as a separate item linked more closely to the public health sciences than community and public health nursing (ACHNE, 1991). Thus, environmental health is considered essential to the education and practice of advanced practice nurses in community health and public health. It should be emphasized, however, that the development of competencies in environmental sciences for generalist and advanced practice nurses who work in traditional settings such as hospitals and long-term-care facilities is also fundamental to their practice in these settings.

### Accreditation and Regulation

The regulation of nursing education and practice is accomplished through a number of credentialing mechanisms. Each mechanism standardizes outcomes (competencies of graduates and practicing nurses) for the assurance of safe delivery of nursing care.

Higher education programs in nursing are accredited by regional accrediting bodies as part of the larger institutional accreditation process. Additionally, schools of nursing seek accreditation from the NLN at the associate degree, diploma, baccalaureate, and master's levels. Within each state, approval for education programs is usually conferred by the state's regulatory board of nursing education content. However, no accrediting body in nursing currently considers environmental health content to be required for the receipt of accreditation.

Official documents of professional nursing organizations endorse the presence of environmental health content in basic and graduate programs. However, accreditation mandates for schools of public health require education in environmental health sciences for graduates of public health programs. Currently, the roles of accrediting bodies and standards in mandating content ensure the visibility of environmental health in schools of public health. Such mechanisms of ensuring an environmental health content bear exploration for the accreditation process in schools of nursing.

## NURSING EDUCATION PATHWAYS

Agreement on the common educational base required for entry into nursing has not yet been achieved (Fagin and Lynaugh, 1992; Oermann, 1994). Oermann argues that the explosion of knowledge, changing health care systems, and community-oriented care demand that nurses be prepared at the baccalaureate level. According to the U.S. Public Health Service (1992), 62 percent of the nurse workforce is prepared at the associate degree and diploma levels, whereas 30 percent of the nursing workforce is prepared at the baccalaureate level. Eight percent is prepared at the master's or doctoral level. When nurses, licensed by the profession, present themselves for employment unprepared for community-based, population-focused practice, the employer has three options:

1. Do not hire, and let positions stay vacant, decreasing capacity for service;

2. Hire and supplement education on the job with formal courses, workshops, and mentoring, with a concurrent investment in more intensive supervision to ensure safe practice; and

3. Hire and decrease job expectations, limiting services to what the nurse is capable of providing, omitting environmental health.

Some or all three of these options have occurred. The aggregate impact is a more limited overall capacity to deliver nursing services that address environmental concerns.

## Basic Nursing Education

In 1994 NLN reported that the number of individuals graduating from the 1,484 registered nursing programs was 80,839—the highest level since 1985. Of these graduates, 65.4 percent (52,896) were from associate degree programs, 26.5 percent (21,415) were from baccalaureate degree programs, and 8 percent (6,528) were from diploma programs (NLN, 1994). However, the projected number of graduates from all three programs by 2000 is expected to shift only because the number of diploma graduates will be reduced to one-third of today's number of diploma graduates. Currently, two-thirds of the registered nurse workforce are graduates of associate degree programs with no curricular experience in public health or environmental health and no clinical experience in these fields (Havens and Stevens, 1990). The major obstacles to including environmental health are lack of curricular time and lack of faculty preparation. It is essential that these barriers be overcome to prepare adequately associate degree nurses to meet the health care demands of individuals, families, and the community.

Professional nursing organizations (e.g., AACN, NLN, ANA, NCSBN [National Council of State Boards of Nursing]) play a major role in influencing the scope of nursing education. Although particular content themes and practical experiences are universal in nursing education (e.g., nursing process, growth, and development) and the graduates of the three types of nursing programs are eligible to take the same licensure exam (National Council Licensure Examination for Registered Nurses [NCLEX]), differences exist among the nursing programs regarding educational preparedness. These differences take the form of inconsistent learning experiences and limited development of competencies in areas of nursing practice essential for the environmental health component of nursing. These competencies include population-focused care, continuity of care, environmental health, health protection, health promotion, disease prevention, and community-based clinical experiences.

Nurses are challenged to engage in activities that promote the *Healthy*

*People 2000* (DHHS, 1990) goals for increasing the time period during which people lead healthy lives, reducing health disparities and achieving access to disease prevention through health promotion, health protection (e.g., improved environmental health), preventive services, and surveillance and data systems. However, continued segmentation or exclusion of nursing competencies in environmental health within general nursing education will not promote nursing's full impact on the goals of *Healthy People 2000*. To be full participants in achieving the health objectives for the nation outlined in the *Healthy People 2000* document, nurses must focus on population-based practice, risk reduction, and preventive services. This focus will require changes in nursing educational preparation, content of nursing practice, and practice settings.

## Graduate Nursing Education

Specialization in nursing occurs at the master's level. In the 1994–1995 school year, there was a 10.7 percent increase in the number of master's degree students enrolled in nursing schools compared with the 1993–1994 school year (AACN, 1994). In 1993, master's programs in nursing numbered 252, with 136 of these offering nurse practitioner programs (NLN, 1994, p. 3).

Master's programs prepare leaders for advanced practice nursing as clinical nurse specialists (CNS), nurse practitioners (NP), certified nurse-midwives (CNM), certified registered nurse anesthetists (CRNA), administrators, teachers, and consultants. Courses in nursing and other science disciplines provide advanced theoretical knowledge, assessment skills, role and leadership development, advanced clinical practice in a selected specialization, and the opportunity to critique and apply nursing theory and research as a scientific base for nursing practice. Increasingly, graduate nursing curricula include core courses such as health assessment, pharmacotherapeutics, health promotion, sociocultural and community health, health economics and policy, theory and ethics, as well as research. Specialty, leadership, and elective courses complete the requirements for the degree.

To date, no standardized curriculum exists for the advanced practice of nursing. However, through regional workshops, the AACN is attempting to define academic instruction, practice, skills, and other essential standard elements of master's-level nursing education. In an AACN interim summary, a core curricular content for all nursing students in master's programs is recommended in the areas of research, economics, ethics and legal issues, health policy, professional role development, nursing theory, and cultural diversity. The areas of consensus on core curricular content for advanced practice nursing programs include advanced health and physical assessment, pathophysiology, and advanced pharmacology. These areas represent the recommendations from participants in three of five AACN workshops.

Increased emphasis has been placed on preparing nurses with advanced practice skills. Numbering nearly 100,000, these individuals have become a significant force in health care delivery (DeAngelis, 1994). The number of advanced practice nurses who graduate annually is predicted to increase by 50 percent by the year 2000, reaching 10,000 annually. Moreover, state laws and federal reimbursement legislation are expanding the authority of advanced practice nurses to practice independently, particularly in underserved rural and inner-city locations (Mundinger, 1994).

The preparation of advanced practice nurses is a particularly fertile arena for addressing the environmental correlates of injury, disease, disability, and the management of acute and chronic illnesses. Advanced practice nurses are also in a strategic role to contribute to and influence the health of the U.S. population. While nurse practitioners primarily provide primary care and clinical nurse specialists are located in hospitals and provide care for more acutely ill persons, the distinctions are blurring. Education at the graduate level must provide the knowledge, skills, and competencies to prepare the APN to effectively incorporate environmental health assessment, risk management, referrals, and risk communication in to practice. Later in this chapter, Table 4.2 lists some graduate-level core courses, the relevant environmental health competencies, and suggested content for each. In addition, as in the basic education table, selected references are included.

### Environmental Health Content in Nursing Education

National sample surveys of baccalaureate and master's nursing programs describing the content of environmental health in curricula were published in the early- to mid-1990s. Rogers (1991) surveyed 423 NLN-accredited schools of nursing with baccalaureate degree programs. Of the 423 schools, 222 (53 percent) responded, and 215 (97 percent) of the respondents indicated that they had some curricular content specific to occupational and environmental health. Information was solicited on eight major content areas within curricula. Four of the eight content areas contained environmental health content specific to the work environment.

Respondents were asked to identify the courses in which this content was taught. Of the respondents, 70 percent–74.4 percent (mean) taught the content in community health nursing courses. Fewer than 15 percent reported teaching it in other courses, such as family nursing or epidemiology courses, or the content was integrated in various courses. Environmental health content in medical-surgical nursing courses was identified by 0.8 percent–6.8 percent (mean) of the respondents and in occupational health nursing courses by 0.6 percent–1.4 percent (mean) of the respondents. The unavailability of a description of the presence and location of the environmental health content by those who did not respond to the survey raises a concern. If the lack of a response (47 percent) reflects an absence of environmental health content, then the environmental health content currently offered in nursing curricula nationwide may be seriously overestimated.

Neufer (1994) points to the incongruity that community health nurses have not been leaders in the field of environmental health, despite their early reliance on Florence Nightingale's emphasis on environment. One indicator of nursing education's emphasis (or lack of it) on environmental health is the content included in current textbooks. In her review of current texts in community health, Neufer identified no text as having all of the factors necessary to address the concepts of environmental health in nursing. She concluded that "although health professionals are becoming more aware of the public health hazards of pollution, community health nurses have not applied their skills in assessing and diagnosing related community health problems." Furthermore, because no text includes all of Neufer's factors, the conclusion follows that these environmental health content areas are not being taught in basic community health courses. Neufer emphasizes that, "the profession must grasp the challenges necessary to promote environmental health" (Neufer, 1994, p. 161).

The importance of environmental health in graduate nursing programs was described in a national sample of 967 leaders in community health nursing service and education, with 588 (61 percent) responding (Selby et al., 1990). Environmental health sciences was a clearly designated target content area for master's-level community health nursing education in the official documents of ANA (1980, 1986), and the Council on Education for Public Health (CEPH, 1986). Environmental health was rank ordered 18–26 of the 43 content areas considered to be core parts of the master's-level community health nursing curriculum by both service and education respondents.

A 1994 University of Minnesota study based on a review of 23 catalogs of schools of nursing with graduate programs in public health or community health nursing found that 17 percent ($N = 4$) required a course in environmental health (Ostwalt and Josten, 1994). In contrast, schools of public health that are accredited by CEPH must provide courses in five content areas, of which environmental health sciences is a requisite area (CEPH, 1986, p. 14). In a recent survey of 187 U.S. nurse practitioner programs, valid responses (90 questionnaires; 48 percent) revealed that more than two-thirds of nurse practitioner program directors believed that greater emphasis should be placed on environmental health. Barriers to change included overcrowded curricula and inadequate faculty preparation. Two factors identified as most likely to facilitate the inclusion of environmental health were, first, the availability of nurse faculty with expertise and, second, access to information resources related to environmental health. Recommendations included (1) the incorporation of environmental health in case history or problem-based instructional designs, (2) inclusion of environmental health risks in patient- or community-assessment learning activities, and (3) use of educational resources such as the *Agency for Toxic Substances and Disease Registry Newsletter* and other training programs (Bellack et al., 1995).

The National Institute for Occupational Safety and Health (NIOSH) provides funding for academic preparation and continuing education in the areas of occupational medicine and nursing, occupational safety, and industrial hygiene. NIOSH has established 14 Educational Resources Center (ERC) programs throughout the country in university settings since 1977 for the education and training of health professionals about occupational health in an interdisciplinary environment. Among the subjects of these programs are risk management and safety, environmental health practice, chemical process hazards, hazardous substance management, and environment and work physiology. The ERCs target occupational health and safety, a subset of the domain of environmental health education (DHHS, 1991).

The Institute of Medicine (IOM) Committee on Enhancing Environmental Health in Nursing Practice conducted 12 focus groups across the country that included leaders of national nursing organizations; practicing nurses prepared from associate, diploma, baccalaureate, master's, and doctoral nursing programs; nurse practitioners; community, public health, and occupational health nurses; nurse educators; and nurse researchers (see Appendix E). Many of the participants illuminated the dilemma of crowded curricula and acknowledged that curricular reform in nursing education was a necessary part of reexamining the competencies required for nurses to deliver health care. Inclusion of environmental health concepts in all basic nursing curricula was recommended as a strategy for reform, as was a shift to context-of-care and community-based practice skills as foundations for nursing interventions. Participants supported the inclusion of general environmental health content and assessment skills in basic nursing courses, with an integration of environmental science as applied to basic and health sciences in pharmacology, physiology, and pathophysiology courses. Some participants voiced concern that environmental assessment was not sufficient and indicated that risk assessment, risk communication, and referrals are necessary skills for all basic nursing graduates. A minority of focus group participants believed that environmental health content should be taught at the graduate level in preparation of specialists for the field. It is unclear however, whether these participants thought that environmental health content should be included at the graduate level only, or that graduate level education should be developed *in addition* to basic nursing education in environmental health.

## MODEL PROGRAM DEVELOPMENT

The philosophical approach of the committee was not to develop a new curriculum, or dictate those elements necessary for basic nursing education. Rather the committee wanted to assist faculty in nursing programs to think about and incorporate environmental health content into existing programs. This section deals with four curricular concerns: (1) to identify the general competencies relevant to environmental health in nursing, (2) to suggest where those competencies may be addressed and integrated into the curriculum, (3) to provide examples of content areas conducive to the inclusion of environmental health in order to link educational activities with the competencies to be achieved, and (4) to suggest resources that will facilitate the teaching of environmental health issues.

### General Competencies

As noted earlier in this chapter, the majority of nurses in the United States are being prepared for registered nurse licensure in associate degree (AD) and hospital diploma programs, with fewer graduating from baccalaureate degree programs. However, it is also known that many nurses with ADs and diplomas are employed in community or public health nursing positions, although community health concepts are not usually included in AD or diploma programs and are not tested in NCLEX. This pattern for testing and employment is not expected to change in the near future.

Based on these facts, the differentiation of environmental health competencies for AD, diploma, and baccalaureate levels may seem an almost futile exercise for nursing education and practice. That is, in nursing education, environmental health content is not required for AD and diploma programs and is included minimally, if at all, in the community health component of baccalaureate programs. None of this content is part of the exam for nursing licensure. Nevertheless, nurses without basic community health nursing preparation are providing many of the community health nursing services in the nation.

Given this somewhat paradoxical situation, in which there is a gap between nursing education and practice, it is important to include environmental health content in as many undergraduate courses as possible. However, rather than detailing the exact environmental health content to be included in each nursing course at every level of nursing education, fairly specific guidelines are provided regarding major environmental health concepts and where these concepts might logically fit in existing nursing curricula. The advantage of this approach is that it allows nursing faculty to integrate environmental health content in an individualized manner based upon faculty expertise, available resources, and the curricular framework specific to each school of nursing. Toward this end, in Table 4.1, the first five courses are ordinarily found in AD and diploma programs, and all the courses are normally part of baccalaureate programs. Environmental health competencies and content examples for each major curricular area are included in Table 4.1 to illustrate the environmental health content that might be appropriate for different levels of basic nursing education. In addition, staff development and continuing education activities are important avenues for increasing the environmental health knowledge and skills of nurses, whatever their training.

The environmental health nursing competency levels of the various types of preparation programs are not easily differentiated. In addition, such a differentiation may not serve a useful purpose at this time because preservice testing does not provide for making this distinction. Further, the level of environmental health competency an individual has attained does not determine employment opportunities or the lack of them for most nurses. The main purpose of including environmental health content in existing curricula at any level is to *enhance* nursing practice in all settings by increasing the awareness and integration of environmental health nursing skills and knowledge in the nursing service provided.

The competencies listed in the box "General Competencies for Nurses" (see Box 3.4 in Chapter 3) are designed for all nurses. However, depending on the level of the educational program, not all competencies will be met to the same degree. The development of learning objectives for the competencies has been left to the discretion of faculty who teach in the various areas to which the competency applies.

## Curriculum Integration Points

*Prerequisites*

Students who enter a baccalaureate nursing program must complete a prenursing curriculum at the same college or university or at another educational institution such as a community college. All types of nursing preparation programs have some prerequisites that must be fulfilled be-

**TABLE 4.1** Basic Nursing Curricula: Courses, Relevant Competencies, Content, Examples, and Suggested References

| Course | Environmental Health Competency[a] | Content Examples | Suggested Resources and References[b] |
|---|---|---|---|
| Physical assessment/ nursing diagnosis | II. Assessment and referral | Environmental history-taking, environmental and occupational health screening, risk communication, home assessment | Appendix D, this volume Taking an Exposure History (ATSDR, 1992) Clues Notebook[c] (Narkunas et al., 1994) IOM (1995) Community as Partner, Chapter 6 (Anderson and McFarlane, 1995) |
| Introduction to concepts/ nursing process | I. Basic knowledge and concepts | Definition of environment, nurse's role in promoting environmental health | Introduction to Nursing, Chapter 5: Environment (Lindberg et al., 1994) Community Health Nursing, Chapter 18: Environmental Health Safety (Stanhope and Lancaster, 1992) Chapter 1 and Appendix A, this volume |
| Medical-surgical (includes gerontology) | II. Assessment and referral III. Advocacy, ethics, and risk communication | Environmentally caused diseases (e.g., cancer, neurologic conditions), referral sources | Priority Health Conditions (Lybarger et al., 1993) Community Health Nursing, Chapter 41: Occupational Health (Stanhope and Lancaster, 1992) |
| Pediatric/maternity or parent, child and family | II. Assessment and referral III. Advocacy, ethics, and risk communication | Childhood toxicants (e.g., lead), sentinel health events (e.g., environmentally induced asthma), reproductive | Nursing Assessment, Chapter 2: Environmental Influences on the Person and Family, Parts III and IV: Developing Person and Family |

| | | | |
|---|---|---|---|
| | | toxicants, home safety, poisoning | (Murray and Zentner, 1989) Nursing in the Community, Chapter 6: Environmental Issues (Bullough and Bullough, 1990) |
| Psychiatry/mental health | II. Assessment and referral<br>III. Advocacy, ethics, and risk communication | Impact of environment on mental health, environmentally induced stress | Community Health Nursing, Chapter 9: Mental Health in the Community (Wold, 1990) Psychiatric Mental Health Nursing (Gary and Kavanagh, 1991) |
| Research | I. Basic knowledge and concepts<br>II. Assessment and referral<br>III. Advocacy, ethics, and risk communication<br>IV. Legislative and regulatory | Environmental health research relevant to nursing | Nursing Research (Polit and Hungler, 1995) |
| Community health | III. Advocacy, ethics, and risk communication<br>IV. Legislative and regulatory | Environmental hazard prevention, recognition, and control; environmental advocacy; environmental justice; ethics; ecology; advocacy; issues (e.g., pollution wastes); environmental health hazards and the nurse (e.g., exposures to tuberculosis or chemotherapeutic agents) | Healthy People: 2000 (DHHS, 1990) Environmental Health in Home Care and Assessment Intervention and Resources (Narkunas et al., 1994) Neufer (1994) Clemen-Stone et al. (1987) Community as Partner (Anderson and McFarlane, 1995) |

continued on next page

**TABLE 4.1** Continued

| Course | Environmental Health Competency[a] | Content Examples | Suggested Resources and References[b] |
|---|---|---|---|
| Leadership/ management | III. Advocacy, ethics, and risk communication<br>IV. Legislative and regulatory | Advocacy and leadership roles to promote environmental health and environmental justice at local, state, and national levels | Perspectives on Family and Community Health, Chapter 21: Leadership and Change in Community Health Nursing Today (Saucier, 1991)<br>Leadership Roles and Management Functions in Nursing (Marquis and Huston, 1992)<br>Community Health Nursing, Chapter 12 (Stanhope and Lancaster, 1992) |

[a]The environmental health competencies are described in detail in Box 3.4 of Chapter 3.
[b]The list of suggested resources and references is not comprehensive; many others are available, as cited in Appendix D.
[c]A rich resource that can be used in numerous courses, the Clues Notebook contains case studies, toxic substances, alerts, and extensive general references and resource information.

fore the student may advance to the nursing curriculum. Ideally, such prerequisite courses would include an introduction to the importance and relevance of environmental health content throughout the nursing education trajectory through basic and advanced preparation.

## Content Areas

The following are examples of how environmental health content can be incorporated into existing courses that are usually considered prerequisites to the professional nursing curriculum:

- include effects of environmental toxicants in a growth and development course;
- include the mechanisms and action of chemicals in the environment that affect health (radon, formaldehyde) in a chemistry course;
- include the role of microorganisms and contaminants in the environment (molds, bacteria) in a microbiology course;
- include the effects of chemicals on organ systems and sentinel environmental illnesses in a pathophysiology course;
- and include the effects of poverty and environmental disasters on mental health in a psychology course.

Both epidemiology and environmental science would be necessary in the curriculum as well if the primary role of the nurse is as a preventionist, as then-president of the NLN Carol Lindeman suggested (Lindeman, 1993).

Although each program uses its own unique framework, the basics of nursing and nursing history are incorporated into courses that cover content in the following prescribed areas: assessment; fundamentals, concepts, and nursing process; care of the medical-surgical patient throughout the life span; care of the pediatric patient; care of the maternity patient (some combine care of the parent and child or call the course family nursing); care of the psychiatric patient and mental health; research; community health; and leadership and management.

## Resources

Table 4.1 presents a list of many of the common courses found in a nursing program; Table 4.2 presents those for graduate nursing. Listed along with each course is an example of suggested environmental health content relevant to the course as well as helpful references and resources addressing that content. The first five courses are part of all basic nursing education and the last three are most often found in baccalaureate programs. Of particular utility as a resource is a recent report from the IOM

**TABLE 4.2** Graduate Nursing Cirricula: Courses, Relevant Competencies, Content Examples and Suggested References

| Course | Environmental Health Competency[a] | Content Example | Suggested Resources and References |
|---|---|---|---|
| Theory and concepts | I. Basic knowledge and concepts | Advanced nursing and other discipline theories related to environmental health | Community Health, Chapter 4: Environmental Health Protection (Green, 1990)<br><br>Exploring Our Environmental Connections (Schuster and Brown, 1994)<br><br>Perspectives on Family and Community Health, Chapter 13: Reconceptualization of the Environment (Saucier, 1991) |
| Advanced health assessment/ pathophysiology/ pharmacology | I. Basic knowledge and concepts<br><br>II. Assessment and referral | Nurse practitioner, community-based prevention and health education | Nursing in the Community, Chapter 6: Environmental Issues (Bullough and Bullough, 1990)<br><br>Primary Care Medicine (Gorall et al., 1995) |
| Advanced practice roles and leadership | I. Basic knowledge and concepts<br><br>II. Assessment and referral<br><br>III. Advocacy, ethics, and risk communication<br><br>IV. Legislative and regulatory | Role development, organizational skills related to specialization | Perspectives on Family and Community Health, Chapter 21: Leadership and Change (Saucier, 1991) |

| Health economics/ policy/global health/ ethics | II. Assessment and referral<br>III. Advocacy, ethics, and risk communication<br>IV. Legislative and regulatory | Economic and political theory, international health, sociocultural concepts, ethics in health care, advocacy | Ethical Dilemmas in Nursing Practice (Davis and Aroskar, 1991) Perspectives on Family and Community Health, Chapter 17 (Saucier, 1991) |
| Research | I. Basic knowledge and concepts<br>II. Assessment and referral<br>III. Advocacy, ethics, and risk communication | Critique of environmental health research, utilization in practice and participation research | Environmental Epidemiology (NRC, 1991) Community as Partner (Anderson and McFarlane, 1995) Measurement in Nursing Research (Waltz et al., 1991) Advanced Nursing and Health Research (McLaughlin and Marasuilo, 1990) |

aThe environmental health competencies are described in detail in Box 3.4 of Chapter 3.

that contains 55 case studies in environmental medicine from the published literature (IOM, 1995). Although the focus in the report is on undergraduate medical education, much of the information presented is directly relevant to nurses.

## METHODS FOR ENHANCING DISSEMINATION OF ENVIRONMENTAL HEALTH CONTENT IN NURSING EDUCATION AT ALL LEVELS

The success of continuing education can be measured by determining whether the quality of education available to nurses positively affects a person's health and care. The dissemination of information to nurses is the first step in changing knowledge, attitudes, and behavior. Dissemination is much more than simply making information available or convincing nurses that it is important. A comprehensive plan for dissemination must consider both the system for distribution and the target of the educational program. Use of existing programs that are targeted to specific needs is a way to begin. One such program is the ATSDR Clues Course, which is designed for community health nurses and environmental health professionals. The course seeks to enhance these health professionals' understanding of the relationship of exposure to hazardous substances to health outcomes, and the role and importance of public health assessments and possible interventions (Narkunas et al., 1994).

### Continuing Nursing Education

Career development in nursing consists of formal academic instruction in a defined program of higher education, licensure, professional continuing education, certification, and advanced practice academic degrees at the master's and doctoral levels. During the late 1960s, nurses nationwide began to identify a need for formal recognition of their participation in continuing education courses. To date, mandatory, approved continuing education for relicensure of registered nurses has been implemented in 22 states (NCSBN, 1994). To ensure safe and professional practice, it is a goal of NCSBN that all states require continuing education for nurses in order to continue their nursing practice. Regardless of how these goals are attained, all nurses should be encouraged to embrace the philosophy of lifelong learning.

The requirement for continuing education brings with it an obligation of the profession to provide the necessary educational programs. This commitment extends to nurses who may work in remote areas, who may not be able to travel to structured classes, or who may have personal or even job-related responsibilities that preclude attendance at workshops or other forms of continuing education. Questions of educational access, replication, and quality are issues for all health professionals and at all levels of education. The application of technological advances in communication is a critical part of the solution.

## Distance Learning

Distance learning is one solution to the lack of access to continuing education. The Commission on Colleges defines distance learning as "that educational process which occurs when instruction is delivered to students physically remote from the main campus, the location or campus of program origin, or the primary resources that support instruction" (Southern Council on Collegiate Education for Nursing, 1994, p. 1).

At the heart of distance learning is the satellite-based information relay, which allows two-way interactive communication in real time. Interactive teleconferencing is approved for continuing education credit by a number of groups throughout the United States. Innovative methods of providing workplace education through satellite telecommunications systems have been proposed, and a growing body of research indicates that both providers and patients view these educational methods as positive and beneficial (Brown et al., 1992; Langford, 1990; Maston and Connover, 1990).

## Media

In recent years, nursing education has undergone a transition involving the integration of concepts in the curriculum rather than the separation of each clinical content area. Increasingly, innovative teaching strategies are being used in nursing programs. Computer technology, interactive video, and other facets of instructional media are now in use in nursing schools, hospitals, and continuing education courses for nurses.

The formal education of children in the United States has experienced rapid integration of computers within the learning environment. Although videodiscs, CD-ROM, and other computer-assisted instruction (CAI) are not used extensively in nursing education, they are gradually being incorporated into many schools of nursing. However, instruction in nursing, especially in basic programs, is still largely dominated by classroom lecture, textbook assignments, and demonstration methods, although teaching nursing students to think critically by analyzing and problem solving has become a basic element of a number of programs and appears to be growing in popularity (Paul, R.W., 1993). Critical thinking is currently a requirement for NLN accreditation.

Although educational technology is a fast-growing, almost explosive area, not all nursing content lends itself to presentation in a multimedia format. The curriculum should drive the technology used, and not the reverse, which sometimes occurs in the frenzied race to incorporate the latest technological innovation. Results of studies on nursing student satisfaction with the classroom use of CAI indicate that the students have mixed feelings. That is, although many students felt positively about the use of CAI in general, not all had favorable attitudes about the use of CAI in their courses (Baldwin et al., 1994; Koch et al., 1990; Lowdermilk and Fishel, 1991; Schare et al., 1991).

There is little doubt that multimedia educational methods will increasingly be adopted as incoming students at all levels are familiar with such technologies. Therefore, the incorporation of computers and interactive video can provide an efficient and cost-effective method of educating both nursing students and practicing nurses. The use of various media in teaching environmental health is also an important way to access the environmental health expertise that is not readily available on campus.

Where more traditional teaching methods are still used, basic and specialty programs can strengthen their community health content as well as acute care content by including environmental health concepts that vitally affect the lives of clients, patients, families, and the communities in which they live and work.

## Interdisciplinary Collaboration

Nursing education is strengthened when students interact with educators who have expertise in environmental health. Nursing faculty with knowledge in environmental and occupational health who can conduct interdisciplinary research are needed to teach students in all nursing programs at all levels. Professionals in such fields as industrial hygiene, toxicology, environmental engineering, and sanitation can augment students' knowledge about environmental health issues. These disciplines are critical for providing a comprehensive approach to the management of environmental health problems concerning individual patients, sites of practice, and the community. It is also important for students to understand the contributions that nurses can make to interdisciplinary efforts in practice, education, and research.

To evaluate effectively the environmental health factors that influence the health of patients, nurses will need to interact and collaborate with specialists in several disciplines. Such interaction may involve knowing the appropriate references in various disciplines and actually consulting with the relevant professionals. Examples of support for interdisciplinary education include the following. First, the IOM study, *The Future of*

*Public Health* (1988), encourages cross-use of faculty among schools on the same or nearby campuses—for example, nursing, public health, medicine, nutrition, and social work—to teach relevant, interdisciplinary content. Second, the W. K. Kellogg Foundation supports a major Community Partnerships Initiative in Health Professions Education and in Public Health that includes interdisciplinary learning and practice as a central feature. Third, the Division of Nursing of DHHS awards funds to schools of nursing and schools of public health to develop dual-degree programs. Faculty can serve as role models for interdisciplinary collaboration by inviting guest faculty from other disciplines to speak about environmental health at schools of nursing, by serving on relevant editorial boards, and by using published materials on environmental health to enhance teaching (see Table 4.3).

## Faculty Development

The NLN recommends that all nurses be prepared to function in a community-based, community-focused health care system. Therefore, faculty must be prepared to meet the shifting demand for knowledge and clinical skills: "Before curriculum reform, then, comes faculty reform" (NLN, 1992, p. 11). Postgraduate programs to expand faculty expertise in population health and interdisciplinary collaboration are endorsed by most national nursing organizations. The population-based approach will require expert knowledge in environmental health sciences, statistics, epidemiology, and public health practice.

Many nurse educators are already familiar with the importance of environmental health. They have some knowledge, depending on their preparation at the graduate level, of environmental hazards (e.g., the oncology nurse is well aware of precautions for handling chemotherapeutic agents) and, as members of the general population, probably share general concerns about environmental quality. Those faculty with particular knowledge, experience, and concerns in environmental health should be identified and nurtured to provide the leadership needed to incorporate the competencies into all educational programs. All nursing faculty need to be involved in this process of incorporation. To strengthen competency development opportunities for nursing students, faculty will require support in their efforts to acquire the necessary knowledge.

Among basic science faculty, such support may mean increasing concern with making courses more clinically relevant as a way to enhance long-term learning, as well as to foster course satisfaction among students. In the process of modifying the basic science curriculum, for example, a faculty member with expertise in environmental health could review the course syllabus and materials with course directors and iden-

**TABLE 4.3** Interdisciplinary Aspects of Environmental Health

| Discipline | Function | Articulation within Nursing Education |
|---|---|---|
| Industrial hygiene | Hazard recognition, evaluation, and control | Community health |
| Toxicology | Toxicity of agents, mechanisms of action, health risks | Pharmacology |
| Safety and injury control | Prevention and control of workplace hazards | Health promotion and disease prevention |
| Ergonomics | Evaluation of worker–environment fit | Health promotion and disease prevention |
| Environmental and occupational medicine | Prevention, recognition, and treatment of environmental and occupational illness and injury | Physical assessment/nursing diagnosis |
| Microbiology | Inspection of eating establishments, water treatment plants, health care facilities | Microbiology/community health |
| Environmental engineering | Assessment of hazardous sites, design of environmental facilities (e.g., water treatment plants) | Community health |
| Environmental chemistry | Analysis of air, soil, and water samples | Community health/pharmacology |
| Epidemiology | Population investigation | Community health |

tify possible points within the course that would be amenable to, and enhanced by the introduction of environmental health examples, case studies, or issues. With some assistance, the course faculty could then incorporate clinically relevant material, as well as opportunities to discuss prevention strategies in lectures or small-group, problem-solving sessions with minimal effort.

Including environmental health content in nursing curricula will require a planned process of change to prepare the faculty and the students for implementation. Schools of nursing may want to assess their previous experience with incorporating major new content areas, for example, physical assessment, for strategies that were successful. Some essential components of any planned change include the following:

- make the new expectations and the rationale for change clear and widely known; allow free and full expressions of feelings and concerns about the change;
- actively discuss ways to address the concerns; show willingness to implement identified strategies for curricular modifications;
- begin developing experts among those faculty who show the most interest and readiness;
- provide opportunities for and reward initiative of those who develop and apply the new content;
- offer mentoring, coaching, and support;
- and continue to reinforce the reason(s) for the change.

Faculty preparation for the changes can be achieved in numerous ways; by presentations at clinical conferences, through formal continuing education programs, in scheduled journal club meetings, and by enrollment in relevant courses that may be available at either home or the nearby institution. Creating regional faculty training institutes in strategically located areas will also promote standardized learning forums in environmental health. Finally, the use of programmed or packaged instruction can enhance faculty skills and knowledge in this area.

Efforts to enhance faculty awareness of environmental health skills and knowledge should focus on faculty who teach in all settings because, as indicated earlier, environmental issues cross all interest and specialty areas. Role modeling as one strategy should be encouraged, and it can work both ways; that is, students involved in environmental issues can sometimes act as catalysts for faculty involvement and vice versa. Faculty role modeling may include active involvement of faculty in environmental issues in the community (including the university or school community), such as advocating for a smoke-free environment or working on a recycling campaign. Even the use of local newspapers to enrich classroom discussion of environmental issues may stimulate further interest in such problems.

Developing faculty to provide leadership regarding environmental health concerns in the curriculum requires a multidimensional approach, as does any change in professional nursing. It is a crucial effort, because the encouragement and support of faculty efforts to improve their own knowledge, skills, and attitudes about environmental health will ultimately result in student efforts being encouraged and supported as well. Examples of faculty development include the following:

• partnership with a practicing nurse who is incorporating environmental health in his or her practice;

• involvement with students in practical projects about environmental concerns;

• a sabbatical (perhaps short-term) spent with environmental science faculty or at a practice site focused on the environment (U.S. or state
Environmental Protection Agency); and

• fellowship awards within the school for faculty who design and
implement a plan for increasing expertise in environmental health.

## ROLE OF FEDERAL, STATE, AND
## LOCAL HEALTH AGENCIES

Various federal, state, and local agencies play a role in monitoring,
supporting, and in some instances, funding the education of nurses. Foundations (e.g., the Pew Commission and the Robert Wood Johnson and
Kellogg foundations) are also visible partners in educating health professionals.

### Federal Agencies

*Health Resources and Services Administration*

On the federal level, the single most influential body affecting nursing education and practice is the Bureau of Health Profession's Division
of Nursing in the Health Resources and Services Administration (HRSA)
of the U.S. Public Health Service, DHHS. The Division of Nursing of
HRSA has a duly constituted National Advisory Council for Nurse Education and Practice (NACNEP) composed of nurses in service and education, members of the public, and nursing students that advise the secretary of DHHS in supporting a broad range of projects such as nursing
education programs for disadvantaged individuals, advanced practice
training grants, primary care preparation, and innovative educational
approaches.

The Division of Nursing of HRSA also undertakes analytical studies,
such as workforce needs and educational-level composition, and the eth-
nic backgrounds, geographic distributions, and other factors related to
nurses and nursing in the United States. On the basis of such data and
projection studies, a major role for NACNEP is in influencing policy for-
mulations and decisions regarding nursing education.

*National Institutes of Health*

The National Institute of Nursing Research as part of the National Institutes of Health (NIH) funds research on the nursing profession and nursing service delivery systems as well as nursing care outcomes. One result of nursing practice and preparation studies is skill mix, which is the use of various levels of nursing knowledge and clinical competence. Other federal agencies, such as the National Institute of Mental Health, National Institute on Aging, the Maternal and Child Health Bureau, the Agency for Health Care Policy and Research, also fund projects involving nurses. These projects can influence nursing education by recommending or making changes in recommended health care practices and nursing care systems.

Many outcomes studies provide evidence for the basis of health policies that affect health care systems, priority setting, and reimbursement to providers, including nurses. However, conclusions based on the results of these studies are oriented more toward the future of nursing than to the basic preparation of nurses. One such conclusion is the need for an increase or decrease in the nursing workforce that is prepared for certain areas such as primary care.

Federal and state environmental policies and agencies help to shape the practice of nursing, but they also have an informal or indirect effect on education programs. For example, if agencies or institutions are hiring only nurses with nurse practitioner certification, educational programs must increase their capacity to teach these students who are requesting this preparation. Otherwise, their enrollments may substantially decrease.

Federal and state agencies remain a critically important resource for all of nursing. For example, environmental epidemiology, especially the study of hazardous waste sites in the United States, determines the nature and limitation of available data on environmental contaminants related to hazardous wastes sites. In addition, federal (e.g., the U.S. Environmental Protection Agency, National Institute of Environmental Health Sciences, and the U.S. Department of Energy) and state agencies are continuously involved in the process of defining which chemicals in the environment are of concern for human health or the levels at which action should be taken to protect human health (NRC, 1991). Such information, although it does not directly influence nursing curricula, can be a source for data and material (e.g., the TRI [Toxic Chemical Release Inventory] database with its user-friendly software) that would be valuable for the enhancement of nursing education, including continuing education programs for nurses in the field.

Federal agencies provide specific "packages" for the education of health professionals. For example, *Clues to Unraveling the Association Between Illness and Environmental Exposure* (Narkunas et al., 1994) is a 7.2 contact-hour program for nurses and environmental health professionals available from the Agency for Toxic Substances and Disease Registry (ATSDR), which is part of DHHS. Other agencies with educational programs include the National Center for Environmental Health and NIOSH (ERCs). The Occupational Safety and Health Administration is another federal agency that is a source of important information. A more complete listing of relevant federal agencies is contained in Appendix D.

## State and Local Agencies

To ensure safe practice, each state board of nursing (or its equivalent) administers a licensing examination. Because each state board of nursing establishes its own scope of practice, it also has the responsibility to monitor the licensed nurse's practice within those parameters, or legal action can be taken. Other state agencies (e.g., health, occupational, and environmental agencies) have no direct jurisdiction over nursing education and practice. Local and state health departments employ nurses to provide services in such areas as public health, maternal-child health, school health, and other targeted areas or to specific populations, and they also serve as clinical practice sites for basic and graduate nursing students. However, funding and revenue sources tend to determine the scope of practice within the boundaries of each state's nursing practice act. For example, if funding for school-based clinics is provided and nurse practitioners are required for primary care, only those nurses who are certified by their state board and/or by the American Nurses Association as nurse practitioners can be employed.[1]

Although local and state environmental agencies can employ nurses, they have less direct or formal contact with nursing education programs. Yet, members of such agencies often serve on advisory committees to nursing education institutions and provide valuable real-world input for curricular improvement and the currency of curricular content. They also serve as resources for technical information and arrange material and sites for student field experience.

Most states have separate health, education, social services, occupational safety and health, environment, consumer affairs, insurance, and other departments that tend to have minimal interagency contact or coordination of services. Therefore, in teaching nurses to practice with a

---

[1]Some states have different (less) requirements for nurse practitioner registration than for ANA certification in specific areas, hence the "and/or." Then, however, they can only work within that specific state. ANA certification is recognized nationally.

comprehensive approach to health that includes physical, mental, social, and environmental health, nursing educators must enable nurses to perform a conceptual integration. That is, they must develop the ability to apply the theoretical knowledge and clinical skills they learn to nursing practice in the way that services are made available to the public. The goal of including environmental health content in all nursing education is to incorporate the concepts into each step of the nursing process.

## METHODS FOR EVALUATING
## EFFECTIVENESS OF CURRICULUM

The evaluation of a nursing education program is an integral part of its development. Sometimes, however, revisions of the curriculum are given considerable attention, whereas evaluation of the modifications is added as an afterthought. Methods of assessing curricular effectiveness depend on the objectives, content, teaching process, and learner. For example, students in an initial nursing preparation program will need to be evaluated on their knowledge and competencies for safe nursing practice. State licensing boards are given this responsibility, and NCLEX is the common testing mechanism. The rationale for including environmental health concepts in basic nursing curricula and in the examination for licensure as a registered nurse has been presented in this chapter.

Because the environment is an increasingly important influence on public health, nurses already in practice should have access to the means for updating their knowledge and skills and applying them in their work settings. Continuing education and distance learning can provide the opportunities to stay current. Problem-based presentations, case studies, vignettes, and pre- and post-tests are means of presenting material as well as of determining the effectiveness of teaching-learning methods and material.

Although preservice licensing tests are administered to assess baseline knowledge, advanced practice certification examinations and second licensure requirements are used to evaluate and/or ensure the acquisition of the additional knowledge and competencies needed for specialized nursing practice. The significance of environmental health in the nursing of individuals, families, and communities makes it imperative that relevant concepts be included and assessed for their currency in all areas of nursing education and practice. It follows that evaluation of the effectiveness of this inclusion by formal means, such as testing, and by informal methods, such as self-assessment of application in practice, is equally important.

A flexible approach to evaluating curricular change is needed when various forms of teaching-learning are used. The commonly used formative (process) and summative (outcome or impact) evaluation methods are useful approaches. Before making any changes, however, an evaluation of the feasibility of curricular revision is a necessary step. What environmental concepts can be included? Where in the nursing program can these concepts be incorporated (e.g., didactic and/or clinical components)? When within the course progression should the content be integrated? (See Table 4.2.) Furthermore, an assessment of the existing curriculum is needed to determine what, if any, environmental health content is already included and where other essential environmental health content might best fit. Faculty who are interested in teaching (or encouraging the teaching of) environmental health must be identified. These faculty can do much to stimulate the interest of students and fellow faculty in a subject by their enthusiasm, example, and commitment.

Another essential step associated with the formative evaluation of curricular modification for the inclusion of environmental content is a form of needs assessment to determine the resources required to implement this activity. Which faculty have the capability and willingness to change the curriculum? How can faculty update or upgrade their own level of knowledge? Are there guest lecturers who would be willing to share their expertise? What resources, both teaching and financial, could be devoted to this activity? What support is needed and available to access teaching tools such as environmental health packets or brochures, audiovisual aids, and computer programs?

A formative (process) evaluation of the curriculum would include the following: review and documentation of the feasibility of incorporating environmental health, what content is incorporated, how it is taught, how frequently, and who is involved. The summative or outcome evaluation is accomplished by measuring student performance on the "General Environmental Health Competencies for Nursing" outlined in Box 3.4 (see Chapter 3). Integrating evaluation activity into existing courses is realistic and amenable to implementation. Systematic planning for the incorporation of evaluation methods in courses within the revised curriculum would result in a relatively comprehensive assessment of program effectiveness with a minimum of added work for the faculty.

Retention of knowledge and actual use of competencies in practice are more difficult to evaluate. Many nursing programs conduct followup surveys of their graduates regarding their employment, field of practice, adequacy of the curriculum, and recommendations for curricular changes. Questions regarding the environmental health content in their particular program and its use in their current practice could be added in order to collect additional evaluation data.

To reiterate, a basic nursing curriculum with enhanced environmental health content in diploma and associate degree programs will be most appropriately evaluated by identifying the specific content additions and then testing for the comprehension, retention, and application of that information. For example, if environmentally caused diseases are included in an existing medical-surgical course in an associate degree or diploma program, the concepts of assessment, referral, and risk communication should be examination items or clinical performance components of a student's evaluation.

For a community health nursing course in a baccalaureate program, the impact of adding content on environmental health policy advocacy should be assessed by evaluating a student's understanding and application of policy and its influence in the didactic portion or in clinical work in a public health agency or community health organization. At the graduate level, evaluations of environmental health content in specialty areas need to be conducted within the master's courses associated with the specialty, such as specific environmental health risks for the elderly in gerontological nursing. As a further illustration, a master's level research course should include epidemiologic environmental health studies, and an evaluation of relevant concepts and critique methods could be done via examination items or an essay.

At this time, licensure tests and specialty certification examinations use a role validation method of test content development. That is, the content of nursing practice in the field largely determines what is tested in the examinations. If nurses do not include environmental health in their practice, it is unrealistic to expect that such content would be covered in the examinations. Therefore, evaluations of curriculum with enhanced environmental health content would currently focus only on the major course(s) in which the additional content has been integrated. The specific method of course and student evaluation used is the prerogative of the faculty responsible for the course as a whole.

Other effects of expanding environmental health content in nursing programs may include changes in faculty awareness and attitudes, increased administrative support for environmental health content, and its inclusion in a variety of educational (e.g., continuing education and distance learning) and health services (e.g., individual or group faculty practices) offered by the school of nursing.

The ultimate objective, and perhaps the most difficult one to measure accurately, is the incorporation of environmental health content into nursing education and practice and the continuous evaluation of how effective it is accomplished in maintaining and promoting the health of individuals, families, and communities. Nonetheless, improvement in the health of all persons by the avoidance or reduction of environmentally induced illness or injury is a worthwhile goal for revising the curricula of nursing education programs.

## RECOMMENDATIONS

To better prepare nurses for the environmental aspects of nursing practice, environmental health curriculum at all levels of nursing education should be enhanced. The committee recognizes that integrating environmental health content into an already crowded curriculum will require creativity on the part of faculty, as well as commitment on the part of educational administrators. Instead of viewing this content as completely new and separate, nursing educators may find ways to emphasize the environmental dimensions of existing courses. Such an integrated approach carries with it, however, the necessity for every faculty member to be knowledgeable about the influences of the environment on health and to actively include environmental content and examples in their teaching. This task is inherently difficult to achieve with a total faculty; a facilitating step would be to have at least one faculty member with particular expertise in environmental health who could champion the curricular adaptations and serve as an internal consultant to other faculty.

The committee also recognizes that most nurses will continue to be educated at differing levels, and that opportunities vary for including environmental health content. Moreover, nurses already in practice will not benefit directly from curricular changes in basic nursing education. Meeting the environmental health content needs of nurses in associate degree and diploma programs, and nurses already in practice requires the development of continuing education opportunities and other kinds of professional support for practitioners. In other words, a range of different strategies will be needed to meet the environmental health training needs of registered nurses (RNs) because of their widely varying employment circumstances.

### Levels of Education

*Recommendation 4.1: Environmental health concepts should be incorporated into all levels of nursing education.*

**Rationale:** Nurses in all settings encounter environmental influences on the health of individuals, families, and communities; therefore, environmental health concepts are essential to the preparation of nurses.

**Strategies for Achieving Recommendation 4.1:**

1. Identify the basic competencies to be included in the development of curricula, as well as the role of advanced practice nurses.

2. Integrate environmental health content into existing prerequisite and basic nursing courses.

3. Develop programs (e.g., faculty fellowships) to increase faculty knowledge and skills in environmental health.

4. Develop model curricula that incorporate environmental health content.

5. Identify and apply educational technology appropriate to the environmental health content and the student population.

## Licensure and Certification Examinations

*Recommendation 4.2: Environmental health content should be included in nursing licensure and certification examinations.*

**Rationale:** Currently, basic nursing licensure and most certification examinations do not explicitly include environmental health content or questions.

### Strategies for Achieving Recommendation 4.2:

1. Develop environmental health test items for nursing licensure and certification examinations.

2. Relay evidence of environmental health content in job expectations and educational programs to state licensing boards and the National Council of State Boards of Nursing (NCSBN).

3. Advocate the inclusion of environmental health in standards for accrediting nursing education (National League for Nursing (NLN) and practice American Nurses Association (ANA).

4. Nurses with expertise in environmental health should participate in advisory committees or boards for certification examinations.

## Environmental Health Disciplines

*Recommendation 4.3: Expertise in various environmental health disciplines should be included in the education of nurses.*

**Rationale:** An interdisciplinary approach is needed to provide health care services required for health conditions caused by environmental factors.

**Strategies for Achieving Recommendation 4.3:**

1. Include professionals from other disciplines associated with environmental health in teaching programs for nurses.

2. Use multidisciplinary and interdisciplinary approaches for field experiences and clinical practice.

3. Identify federal, state, and local environmental health resources.

## Lifelong Learning

*Recommendation 4.4: Environmental health content should be an integral part of lifelong learning and continuing education for nurses.*

**Rationale:** With rapid changes occurring in environmental influences on health, keeping current is an important responsibility of all nurses.

**Strategies for Achieving Recommendation 4.4:**

1. Existing educational materials (e.g., ATSDR Case Studies, CLUES program, and related IOM reports) should be disseminated more broadly.

2. Nurses should participate in educational programs of professional organizations that include environmental health content.

3. Professional journals should publish more articles on environmental health.

4. Incorporate environmental health content in computer-based professional education programs.

## Educational Resources and Opportunities

*Recommendation 4.5: Professional associations, public agencies, and private organizations should provide more resources and educational opportunities to enhance environmental health in nursing practice.*

**Rationale:** Nurses will need a basic knowledge of environmental health concepts, resources, and intervention strategies to identify and successfully act upon environmental health problems. However opportunities for nurses to learn about environmentally related illnesses are severely limited because of such factors as a lack of support for continuing education, a lack of nursing faculty who are qualified to teach such content, a lack of support for faculty and program development, and a lack of institutional support for their attendance at such programs.

**Strategies for Achieving Recommendation 4.5:**

1. Encourage professional associations to provide continuing education concerning environmental health, particularly associations that represent specialists in community and public health, pediatrics, occupational health, reproductive health, and primary care.

2. Provide funding from public and private agencies to provide educational opportunities for nurses at all levels to enhance their knowledge of environmental concepts.

3. Promote institutional support for continuing education in environmental health for (a) nurses to attend such programs, and (b) schools of nursing to develop programs on the topic of environmental health.

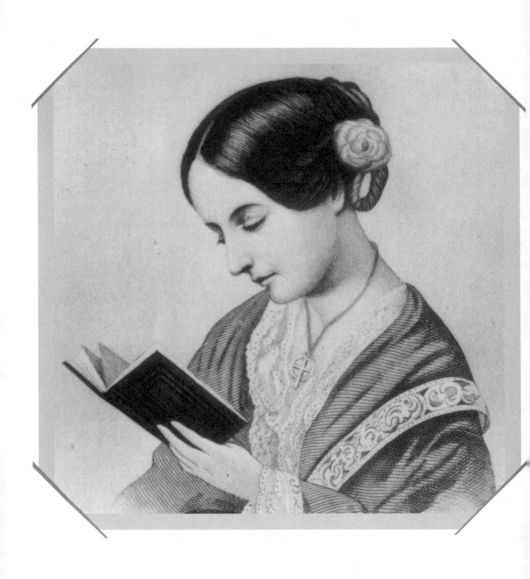

*Florence Nightingale as she appeared at the time of the Crimean War.*

*Engraving by G.E. Perine & Co. from a crayon drawing (no date).*
*Property of Duke University Medical Center Library,*
*History of Medicine Collections, Durham, NC.*

# 5

# Nursing Research

*In dwelling upon the vital importance of sound observation, it must never be lost sight of what observation is for. It is not for the sake of piling up miscellaneous information or curious facts, but for the sake of saving life and increasing health and comfort.*

—Florence Nightingale, 1860, p. 125

*Population growth, urbanization, new energy sources, advanced technology, industrialization, and modern agricultural methods have enabled unprecedented progress. At the same time, they have created hazards to human health that are dramatically different from hazards of the past. Synthetic chemicals, new sources of toxic substances, and naturally occurring radiation are distributed throughout the environment. The potential risks from many of these agents were initially either unrecognized, underestimated, or accepted as inevitable and minor in comparison to the benefits of modernization and economic growth. Public awareness and perceptions have changed. Extensive research programs, carried out in public health and environmental agencies, are under way to determine the potential harmful effects of chemical agents on the environment and health.*

—*Healthy People 2000* (DHHS, 1990, p. 312)

Implicit in the *Healthy People 2000* objectives is the recognition that within the next decade, research is certain to provide a better understanding of the relationship between exposure to environmental hazards and adverse health outcomes. Nursing research could also be expanded to address the nature of hazards in the physical environment and their impact on human health.

The impact of the human-physical environment interaction on the health of individuals and of all people has been an enduring theme in the development of the discipline and science of nursing (Donaldson and Crowley, 1978). Indeed, in the early nineteenth century Florence Nightingale, a pioneer in the development of nursing science, emphasized that the nature and quality of a patient's physical environment are determinants of the patient's recovery of health. A major therapeutic function of nurses was to control the physical environment (Nightingale, 1860). However, the centrality of studies of the physical environment to nursing science has been lessened by the emergence of competing realms, such as studies that address other types of human relationships (e.g., social and nurse-client) and their impact on human health. One of the challenges to nursing presented by the *Healthy People 2000* report is to reemphasize the importance of research related to physical environmental hazards and the health of humans.

## NURSING RESEARCH PERSPECTIVE

Nursing research emanated from and continues to develop because of a societal mandate and demand for professional nursing services. As a branch of disciplinary knowledge, nursing is a professional rather than an academic discipline (Donaldson, 1995; Donaldson and Crowley, 1978), and nursing research reflects the profession's focus on the health status and care of individuals and populations.

According to the National Institute for Nursing Research, National Institutes of Health (established in 1993 to supersede the National Center for Nursing Research [National Center for Nursing Research, 1993, p. 5]):

> Nursing is the discipline associated with the science and art of care-giving. Although all health professionals care about those to whom they provide services, actual acts of care-giving in health and illness are most frequently performed by nurses. The nursing discipline grew out of public demand for educated, formal caregivers devoted to the public good. Throughout its history, nursing has espoused the idea that care-giving during health and illness must be organized around individuals, families, and communities rather than diseases (Lynaugh and Fagin, 1988). Nursing also recognizes the effect of culture in shaping the definition of health and illness and interpreting human responses to physiological and biological changes.

The nursing research perspective focuses on understanding the biological and behavioral elements of human health rather than on elucidating diseases and their treatment or cure. Understanding the complex relationship between human behavior and the physical and biological environmental hazards with the aim of assisting in bringing about the requisite changes in societal action and human behavior is the major focus of nursing in environmental health. The knowledge generated from nursing research provides information on how humans achieve health, respond to threats to their health, and cope with disease, as well as how to treat disease. In nursing research the conceptualization of *human* (either individual or collective) is holistic, and a priority is the preservation of human autonomy in the achievement of health (Donaldson, 1995; Gortner,

1990). Thus, in the area of environmental health, nursing research addresses (1) human responses to potential and real environmental hazards and (2) interventions directed toward preventing exposure to environmental hazards (primary intervention), limiting exposure to the hazards (secondary intervention), and treating or rehabilitating individuals exposed to environmental hazards (tertiary intervention). Nursing research also addresses the quality and safety of the physical environment from the perspective of how humans interact with their environment in their general pattern of living. An example of this type of research is the work-related enhancement of person-environment compatibility by reducing ambient stresses such as noise and sound levels (Topf, 1994). Nursing research is also directed toward quality control of the human physical environment and public policy related to that goal. Nursing research thus spans from the individual human biological (e.g., physical symptoms of lead poisoning) and behavioral (e.g., ingestion of paint chips) responses to collective or group behavior (e.g., community-based efforts or regulatory policy to remove a hazard) in the area of environmental health.

## MULTIDISCIPLINARY RESEARCH BASE FOR NURSING PRACTICE

As a profession, nursing's highest priority is professional practice that is research based and scholarly. The significant changes that are occurring in the scope of nursing clinical practice and the curricula of the professional educational programs require a supporting knowledge base. If the area of environmental health is to be incorporated into all realms of nursing practice, an appropriately conceptualized knowledge base must be available and continually expanded. In clinical practice, nurses provide service in a wide variety of settings that are significant to humans (e.g., health care facilities, home, workplace, school, and community). Nurses plan their intervention strategies in the context of the setting, the social network, and the resources of the client.

Knowledge essential to this clinical practice is that derived from nursing research as well as the more traditional areas of environmental health research such as human disease manifestation, risk assessment, and risk management. Nurses in clinical practice need to have knowledge of these traditional realms to recognize and identify hazards, but they also must know how to control the quality of the physical environment and to effect change in human behavior (whether it be an individual's lifestyle or policy-making) to help individuals avoid, reduce, or eliminate environmental hazards. Nurses also participate in treating humans affected by these hazards. For example, radioactive contamination of soil has adverse effects on the health of an individual (e.g., increased risk of cancer, adverse reproductive effects) and community health (e.g., contaminated food and water supplies). Studying this hazard and treating humans affected by this hazard are major challenges that should be addressed by many disciplines and professions, including nursing. Thus, research and clinical practice in environmental health best serve societal health when they are approached from an interdisciplinary perspective in both research and practice.

## REVIEW OF NURSING RESEARCH IN
## ENVIRONMENTAL HEALTH

The committee conducted a review of recently funded research projects and recently published research reports to ascertain the scope and general nature of nursing research activity in environmental health. For the purposes of the review, nursing research grants were defined as environmental health and occupational health projects if they could be directly related to clinical nursing practice and to the discipline of nursing (i.e., nurse principal investigator and funded by a nursing organization or conducted in a unit of higher education with a formal professional nursing education program, such as a school of public health). In conducting the literature search, research reports were categorized as nursing research if they were published in a nursing journal and pertained directly to nursing practice, regardless of whether the author was a nurse.

The databases surveyed for funded research projects were broad. They were chosen with the intention of capturing the majority of the funded projects in the general area of environmental and occupational health and included a survey of those professional and private research organizations known to fund nursing research (Table 5.1). Similarly, the survey of research reports in the published literature was broad and included surveys of large databases such as MEDLINE and CINAHL to capture as much nursing research as possible in the area of environmental and occupational health (Table 5.2). The search parameters for the various databases surveyed are given in Tables 5.1 and 5.2. Note that the funded projects identified as nursing research all had a nurse as a principal investigator and were funded by a nursing organization or conducted in a unit of higher education with a formal professional nursing program, such as a school of public health. For those funded grants and published reports identified as nursing research in environmental and occupational health in Tables 5.1 (21 grants) and 5.2 (14 papers), an additional content analysis was performed as shown in Table 5.3. The coded study characteristics and categories used in this content analysis of each project or report are given in Table 5.3; note that the published papers analyzed for Table 5.3

**TABLE 5.1** Recently Funded Research Grants from the Government and Professional or Private Research Organizations Related to Environmental Health Content in Nursing

| Databases Surveyed for Funded Research | Parameters | No. of Citations | No. of Nursing Research Grants Directly Related to Environmental Health |
|---|---|---|---|
| **Government Agencies** | | | |
| Department of Defense | Grants involving nurses, 1993–1994 | 30 | 2 |
| National Institute of Environmental Health Sciences | Grants active in 1994 | 737 | 0 |
| National Institute of Justice | Grants active in 1993 | 98 | 0 |
| National Institute for Nursing Research | Grants active in 1993 | 500 | 6 |
| National Institute for Occupational Safety and Health | Grants involving nurses, 1990–1994 | 2 | 1 |
| **Subtotal** | | 1,367 | 9 |
| **Professional or Private Research Organizations** | | | |
| American Cancer Society | All environmentally related grants, 1990–1993 | 345 | 0 |
| American Heart Association | All awards to individuals, 1992–1993 | 2,476 | 0 |
| American Association of Occupational Health Nurses | Environmentally related research, 1990–1994 | 8 | 8 |
| American Nurses Foundation | All grants, 1990–1993 | 109 | 1 |
| Association of Women's Health, Obstetrics and Neonatology | All grants, 1990–1994 | 24 | 0 |
| Oncology Nursing Society | All grants, 1990–1994 | 95 | 0 |
| Sigma Theta Tau International | All grants, 1990–1993 | 68 | 3 |
| **Subtotal** | | 3,125 | 12 |
| **TOTAL** | | 4,492 | 21 |

**TABLE 5.2** Recently Published Research Reports Related to
Environmental Health in Nursing

| Literature Databases Surveyed | Parameters | No. of Citations | No. of Nursing Research Reports Directly Related to Environmental Health |
|---|---|---|---|
| CINAHL Medline ERIC NTIS Conference   Paper Index | Terms used include:   community health nursing,   maternal or child health   and nursing, nursing and   environment, occupational   health nursing, pediatric   nursing, and public health   nursing (1990–July 1994) | 1,098 | 14 |

did not have to have a nurse principal investigator or a nursing organization affiliated with the principal investigator.

For all of the survey data collection and content analysis of individual research projects, two committee members developed and pilot tested a coding sheet to test the reliability and the completeness of the data collected. All discrepancies in coding between coders were resolved by consensus.

### Results of Review

Results of the survey of funding agencies are reported in Table 5.1. The total pool of grants reviewed was large (4,492), but only a small proportion (21 of 4,492, or 0.5 percent) was identified as nursing research in environmental or occupational health. Similarly, only a small proportion (14 of 1,098, or 1.3 percent) of the relevant research literature was in the area of nursing research in environmental or occupational health (Table 5.2). Government agencies, professional nursing organizations, and private organizations participated in funding of the grants and published research articles.

The results of the content analysis of the 35 projects and publications identified as nursing research in environmental or occupational health are displayed in Table 5.3. The data reported in Table 5.3 reflect a high proportion (94.3 percent) of nurse principal investigators, which was somewhat expected, since all of the funded grants ($n = 21$) had a requirement of a nurse principal investigator. But even in the review of the literature, 12 of the 14 (85 percent) published papers that were catego-

**TABLE 5.3** Characteristics of Nursing Research in Environmental or Occupational Health: 1990–1994 ($n$ = 35 grants and published reports from Tables 5.1 and 5.2)

| Characteristics of Nursing Research | Description of Characteristic | % of Nursing Research ($n$) |
|---|---|---|
| Investigator | Nurse | 94.3 (33) |
| | Other | 5.7 (2) |
| Affiliation of principal investigator | School of nursing | 48.6 (17) |
| | Corporate | 20.0 (7) |
| | Unknown | 14.3 (5) |
| | Other university | 11.4 (4) |
| | Government | 5.7 (2) |
| Funding source | None or not noted | 22.9 (8) |
| | American Association of Occupational Health Nurses | 22.9 (8) |
| | National Institute for Nursing Research | 17.1 (6) |
| | Emergency Room Nursing Foundation | 8.6 (3) |
| | Sigma Theta Tau International | 8.6 (3) |
| | Department of Defense | 5.7 (2) |
| | Occupational Safety and Health Administration | 5.7 (2) |
| | American Nurses Foundation | 2.8 (1) |
| | Centers for Disease Control and Prevention | 2.8 (1) |
| | National Institute for Occupational Safety and Health | 2.8 (1) |
| Funding amount | Unknown | 60.0 (21) |
| | <$1,000 | 14.3 (5) |
| | $1,000–$50,000 | 14.3 (5) |
| | $50,000–$100,000 | 2.8 (1) |
| | >$100,000 | 5.7 (2) |
| | None | 2.8 (1) |
| Focus | Occupational | 91.4 (32) |
| | Environmental | 8.6 (3) |
| Topics | Populations at risk | 74.3 (26) |
| | Disease or condition | 22.9 (8) |
| | Prevention | 22.9 (8) |
| | Particular hazard | 20.0 (7) |
| | Education | 14.3 (5) |
| | Policy | 11.4 (4) |
| Population studied | Industrial workers | 22.9 (8) |
| | Nurses | 20.0 (7) |
| | Office/municipal workers | 20.0 (7) |
| | Agricultural workers | 17.1 (6) |
| | Pregnant women/new mothers | 8.6 (3) |
| | Neonates | 5.7 (2) |
| | Disabled | 2.8 (1) |
| | Rats | 2.8 (1) |

continued on next page

**TABLE 5.3** Continued

| Characteristics of Nursing Research | Description of Characteristic | % of Nursing Research ($n$) |
|---|---|---|
| Health hazards/ conditions studied | General health | 28.6 (10) |
| | Musculoskeletal | 17.1 (6) |
| | Hearing impairment | 11.4 (4) |
| | Accidents | 8.6 (3) |
| | Lead exposure | 2.8 (1) |
| | Conjunctivitis | 2.8 (1) |
| | Natural disasters | 2.8 (1) |
| | Disability | 2.8 (1) |
| | Pesticides | 2.8 (1) |
| Study designs | Descriptive | 80.0 (28) |
| | Intervention/experimental | 20.0 (7) |

rized as nursing research in environmental or occupational health were authored by nurses. Most (48.6 percent) of the principal investigators of the research grants and published papers were affiliated with schools of nursing; other nonnursing units of universities represented 11.4 percent of the principal investigators, making institutions of higher education the primary source of nursing research in environmental or occupational health. Corporations were affiliated with 20 percent of the research.

The data in Table 5.3 also indicate that there are funding sources for nursing research in environmental health, such as the Centers for Disease Control and Prevention (CDC), Emergency Room Nursing Foundation, and the Occupational Health and Safety Administration (OSHA) that were not included in the databases that were searched for funded grants (Table 5.1). The focus of the grants and published reports (Table 5.3) was primarily occupational health (91.4 percent), the topics, subject groups, and health hazards or conditions were broad, and the design of the research projects was predominantly descriptive (80 percent).

## Discussion of Review

On the basis of the survey results, there is, in general, a dearth of research in environmental or occupational health related to the practice of nursing. Nursing research represents an extremely small component of the portfolio of funded research of the agencies and organizations polled (Table 5.1; 9 of 1,367, or 0.6 percent, of government grants and 12 of 3,124, or 0.4 percent, of grants from professional and private research organizations). The reason for this underrepresentation of nursing research in environmental or occupational health was not explored, but it likely reflects a very small pool of nurse researchers in general. Thus, nurse researchers and nursing research in the area of environmental or occupational health are underrepresented in terms of numbers and activity, respectively.

Nonnurse investigators in the area of environmental or occupational health do not appear to be conducting studies directly related to the knowledge base for nursing practice. Expansion of the research directly related to the practice of nurses in the area of environmental or occupational health is most likely to be accomplished by expanding the research conducted by nurse investigators.

Currently, nurse principal investigators in the area of environmental and occupational health identified in the survey are primarily affiliated with schools of nursing (48.6 percent; Table 5.3). Of interest is that the principal nurse investigators in corporate settings identified in the review (Table 5.3) make up a higher proportion (20 percent) than the proportion in other, nonnursing university units (11.4 percent), for example in schools of public health. This finding is most likely a reflection of the predominant occupational health focus of the studies captured as part of the survey of the literature (91.4 percent; Table 5.3). Schools of nursing and universities are the administrative homes for the majority of the nurse investigators in environmental or occupational health. However, there is evidence that the private sector is active in nursing research.

The scope of the research studies surveyed (grants and published papers) seems to be broad in terms of topics, subject groups, and health hazards or conditions. In contrast, the type of design (i.e., descriptive studies) and total funding for nursing research appear to be limited. Current nursing research in the area of environmental or occupational health appears to be predominantly descriptive rather than clinical studies employing experimental or other nonexplorative designs. This is a limitation because the application of knowledge to practice generally follows clinical intervention studies. The reason for the preponderance of descriptive nursing research studies is not known, but descriptive work usually signifies a research realm in which the problems and variables are not well defined or little is known about the area. In other words, to conduct research that can serve as a basis for clinical nursing practice in environmental or occupational health, it may be necessary to conduct some descriptive studies to identify appropriate and valid biobehavioral models from which nursing interventions could emanate. However, the highly descriptive research found in the survey might also reflect an inadequate focus of the research on clinical intervention strategies for nurses, even though it is conducted by nurse investigators. It is difficult to ascertain information regarding the nurse's role in multidisciplinary team research where the nurse is not a co-investigator.

Regardless of the reason for the predominantly descriptive nature of the work, it is clear that scant research supports the clinical practice of nursing in environmental or occupational health. Because nursing, like the other health professions, strives to base its clinical practice and educational programs on knowledge generated from research, the volume of relevant clinical research in environmental health must be increased to support nursing practice in this area. To generate an adequate knowledge base to support nursing practice in environmental or occupational health, the numbers of nurse researchers and funded projects must be increased, and the design of the work must be broadened to include experimental and intervention studies.

## MEETING THE NEED FOR NURSING RESEARCH IN ENVIRONMENTAL HEALTH

### Development of the Cadre of Nurse Researchers

Nurses at all educational levels can contribute to the research enterprise in meaningful ways, be it problem identification, risk assessment, investigation, data analysis, dissemination of knowledge, research utilization, policy formulation, or risk communication. However, nurses at the doctoral level must be prepared to guide these investigations. Because of their unique access to people in multiple settings, nurses are essential for identifying researchable problems and questions. For example, maternal and child health nurses could be continuously screening children who may have been exposed to residential lead-based paint or pesticides on farms; emergency room nurses could attempt to decipher how individuals are exposed to toxic wastes or environmental poisons; occupational health nurses could be screening for the vast array of workplace exposures resulting in illness and injury such as reproductive toxicity, cancer, neurological dysfunction, and musculoskeletal disorders; and pediatric nurses could be linking childhood illnesses to toxins transported from a parent's workplace to the home.

Nurses working in community health, especially those in inner-city and rural settings, have a key role in environmental health. Some nurses in community-based practice are involved in identifying group patterns of illnesses and sentinel health events that may have their origins in environmental exposures (Lipscomb, 1994b; Rogers, 1994). For example, a draft U.S. Environmental Protection Agency (EPA) report stated that epidemiological studies of extremely low-frequency electromagnetic field exposures and leukemia, lymphoma, and cancers of the nervous system among children and workers show a consistent pattern of response that suggests but does not prove a causal link (EPA, 1990). This conclusion is supported by several epidemiological investigations that have shown higher rates of brain tumors and leukemia among children who lived near high-distribution lines (Savitz, 1988); greater risk for brain cancer in workers with high levels of exposure to electromagnetic radiation (Savitz and Loomis, 1995); developmental delays and miscarriages from exposure to electric blankets and ceiling cable heating systems (Wertheimer and Leeper, 1986, 1989); and a possible link between male breast cancer and electromagnetic field exposure in telephone linemen (Demers, 1990; Matanowski et al., 1989). Clearly, public health or community health nurses could be involved in identifying and investigating these types of problems.

Nurses who complete a thesis as part of their masters degree requirements are prepared to conduct preliminary or pilot studies related to their specialties, work settings, or problems identified through their clinical practice. For example, community health nursing programs identify, collect, and analyze population-based data. However, although research is a component of their practice, it is not the focus of their professional responsibilities. As in the other health professions and sciences, the leaders and principal investigators of nursing research are best prepared in educational programs that require a dissertation in either the field of nursing or other disciplines. The graduate degrees in nursing that correspond to this preparation are the PhD, DNS, DNSc, and DSN (Doctor of Nursing Science). Although research is one component of the curriculum in baccalaureate and master's programs in nursing, the purpose of these non-doctoral-level programs is to prepare nurses to apply research and to act as participants in the research process. The preparation of independent investigators is the domain of the graduate-level doctoral programs. Currently there are 49 PhD programs and 11 DNS/DNSc/DSN programs in institutions of higher education in the United States (American Association of Colleges of Nursing [AACN] 1994–1995 Enrollment and Graduations Baccalaureate and Graduate Programs in Nursing). Postdoctoral nursing research programs are also available at 12 institutions. Existing nurse researchers might use postdoctoral programs in nursing or environmental health-related sciences (e.g., toxicology and public health) to gain expertise in conducting research in environmental health. Because of the interdisciplinary nature of environmental health, educational programs and mentorships involved in interdisciplinary research are desirable. Additionally, nurses with doctorates in related environmental health sciences may be particularly helpful in integrating nursing research and facilitating the interdisciplinary nature of research.

Solutions to the problems and questions presented by the complex interaction between humans and their environment generally require the collaboration of investigators in several disciplines. Nursing has a place in these interdisciplinary endeavors. Fostering interdisciplinary research, in which nurses interact to identify and study environmental topics of concern, will result in a wide range of contributions that can be used to solve problems. Moreover, the fairly recent revolution in academic nursing research was created, above all, by scientists pursuing not only support for their own investigations, but also opportunities to participate in exciting science. To benefit from the valuable observations and powers of reasoning of those nurse researchers with firsthand knowledge of humans in their environments, communication with the broad research community, both intradisciplinary and interdisciplinary, must be improved. The NIOSH-sponsored Educational Resource Centers (see Chapter 4) can be a tremendous resource to researchers in environmental health because of their multidisciplinary nature.

The number of openings for students in existing doctoral programs in nursing is limited, and environmental health is not a current focus in these programs. Thus, there are major challenges to increasing the cadre of nurse researchers in environmental health. Stimuli are needed to expand doctoral programs in nursing and to redirect the programmatic offerings to emphasize research in environmental health. Implicit in such efforts is support for faculty research programs in environmental health and for researchers who can mentor doctoral and postdoctoral students. There is also value in nurses seeking doctorates in nonnursing disciplines (e.g., toxicology and epidemiology).

The interaction of environmental factors associated with acute and chronic illness, health promotion, and disease prevention are important foci of nursing research to improve the health of the community and patient care. To take advantage of the rapid changes taking place in the environmental sciences and to explore these environmental linkages, training and career development resources should be focused on the areas of environmental science that underlie and influence nursing practice (e.g., human response to environmental exposures and conditions). Thus, there is a need for research training and career development in the environmental sciences to (1) develop a cadre of nurse scientists with research training at the predoctoral and postdoctoral levels in environmental science and nursing science and (2) enhance the knowledge base of midcareer nurses with doctorates whose research relates to or might be redirected to environmental sciences.

The overall goal of a training initiative would be to increase the number of nurse researchers in the environmental sciences who are prepared to explore the environmental linkages to nursing practice and research as they affect the public's health. To accomplish this goal, it is important that applicants for research funding include a nurse scientist as cosponsor when the sponsoring environmental scientist (i.e., mentors) does not have a nursing degree. Training and career development programs could provide opportunities for nurses to conduct supervised clinical and basic research at the interface between nursing and at least one of the traditional environmental disciplines. The academic, clinical, and laboratory environments could facilitate growth and development for promising students, new research scientists, and midcareer scientists. Important elements of training would include, for example, ongoing interactive departmental seminars; a faculty well published in refereed journals; and an interactive, interdisciplinary research team funded by multiple sources. This type of training opportunity links research and graduate education—the defining strength of academic research and the education enterprise.

The National Institute for Nursing Research is committed to promoting the development of a career trajectory for research training of nurse investigators. The purpose of the trajectory is to operationalize the philosophical stance that research training is a career commitment. Such a trajectory allows researchers to remain updated and in the forefront of the content and methodologies of their scientific fields. A series of award mechanisms are available to facilitate research training and career development.

### Current Priorities of Funding Sources for Nursing Research

Nursing research and research education in environmental and occupational health sciences have several sources of interdisciplinary support. Those organizations most likely to be interested in environmental health and nursing are listed in Table 5.1 and were included in the survey. However, it is also apparent from the survey that there is some private-sector corporate funding for nursing research. The potential of this funding source has not been explored.

### Sigma Theta Tau International

Since 1992 Sigma Theta Tau International (STTI) has engaged in joint endeavors with several specialty organizations to fund collaborative research projects. Rogers (1994) reported on such efforts between STTI and the American Association of Critical Care Nurses, STTI and the Oncology Nursing Society, STTI and the Emergency Nurses Association, and STTI and the American Association of Diabetes Educators, whereby research projects are jointly funded and overall administrative coordination is handled by the specialty organization. The participating organizations jointly recognize the award recipients.

*National Institute for Nursing Research, National Institutes of Health*

The National Institute for Nursing Research (NINR) and the National Institute of Environmental Health Sciences (NIEHS) have announced their interest in receiving individual and institutional National Research Service Award (NRSA) applications for support of training at the pre- and postdoctoral levels for nurses interested in pursuing research careers combining environmental health and nursing sciences. Applications for predoctoral awards will be considered only by NINR. The purpose is to provide a cadre of nurse investigators who can apply the principles of clinical nursing research to environmental health research problems and to achieve the health promotion and disease prevention objectives of *Healthy People 2000* (DHHS, 1990).

Targeted NRSA fellowships in environmental sciences must focus on environmental science development, advanced clinical science development, and supervised research training experience. Applicants must integrate an area of environmental theory with a relevant nursing problem. It is necessary that the sponsor be an environmental nurse scientist or an environmental scientist with a nurse scientist as cosponsor. The following are currently available NRSA fellowships:

• The predoctoral environmental science fellowship is designed to provide predoctoral nurses with supervised clinical or basic environmental research training leading to the PhD. Applicants must be registered nurses.

• The postdoctoral environmental science fellowship is designed to provide postdoctoral research training to nurse scientists who wish to refine their research interests, initiate independent research programs, and gain depth of knowledge in their clinical or basic environmental research area. To prepare scientists to explore the environmental underpinnings of nursing practice and research, applicants must integrate environmental science with a nursing problem or a clinical practice issue. Priority status will be given to nurses with doctorates who submit a successful postdoctoral NRSA application, which would enable continued training without a break between doctoral and postdoctoral programs. To ensure maximum growth and development as a research scientist and to increase the integration of new theories and ideas, postdoctoral fellows are advised to choose universities or departments other than the site of their doctoral training.

• The senior biological science fellowship award provides advanced training for experienced nurse scientists (with at least 7 years of relevant research or experience beyond the doctoral level). These awards are designed to enable nurse scientists to take time off from their regular professional responsibilities to make major changes in the direction of their research careers or to broaden their scientific backgrounds by acquiring new research capabilities. This award is directed at nurse researchers who are well prepared in environmental science and who desire to learn new methodologies and techniques. For example, a nurse scientist might combine sabbatical time with senior biological science fellowship funding.

NINR also has available the full menu of National Institutes of Health-type research (e.g., investigator-initiated R01) and training awards (K type) for investigator-initiated projects, which could include environmental health. One such opportunity, the Exploratory Center Award mechanism (e.g., P20) has worked well for establishing centers of excellence in multidisciplinary research in various realms of nursing science.

## National Institute for Occupational Safety and Health

In recent years the National Institute for Occupational Safety and Health (NIOSH) began to fund nursing research and nursing research training originally related to the 10 leading causes of morbidity and mortality that are biomedical in origin. The effort to emphasize the linkage of nursing research to national priorities gives graduate students more opportunities to participate in interdisciplinary research that is relevant to occupational health, safety, and related issues. Students thereby gain increased experience working in multidisciplinary and often multisectional groups on projects designed to highlight connections between new knowledge and the health and well-being of society.

NIOSH offers a variety of research awards that are frequently related to the cause and prevention of leading work-related problems identified by NIOSH. This source provides a specific funding avenue for nurses who desire to investigate occupational health, safety, and related issues.

## American Association of Occupational Health Nurses

The American Association of Occupational Health Nurses (AAOHN) offers competitive annual awards to promote and recognize research and innovative projects that focus on issues and problems within occupational health nursing. Research priorities established by AAOHN identify a wide range of researchable topics for occupational health nursing investigations.

## RECOMMENDATIONS

### Scope of Nursing Research in Environmental Health

*Recommendation 5.1: Multidisciplinary and interdisciplinary research endeavors should be developed and implemented to build the knowledge base for nursing practice in environmental health.*

**Rationale:** Despite the match of the nursing research perspective with the realm of environmental health, there is a dearth of research to support environmental health in clinical nursing practice. Furthermore, designs for nursing research projects in environmental health are of inadequate methodological depth, and are primarily descriptive.

**Strategies for Achieving Recommendation 5.1:**

1. Establish multidisciplinary environmental health training grants that include content in physical, biological, and behavioral sciences relevant to nursing practice.

2. Provide incentives for multidisciplinary mentorship for pre- and postdoctoral research fellowships that include nursing research.

3. Provide incentives to include a nursing research component in environmental health program projects.

4. Establish mechanisms for nurse researchers to interact with and access the resources of the existing National Institute for Occupational Safety and Health's Educational Resource Centers and the National Institute of Environmental Sciences' Environmental Health Centers.

5. Use existing mechanisms for establishing multidisciplinary centers of research excellence, such as the NIH Exploratory Center Award (P20), to develop sites for nursing research in environmental health.

6. Individual nurse researchers should seek collaborative research opportunities in environmental health.

7. Include nurses as members of editorial boards and institutional review boards (IRBs).

### Availability of Researchers

*Recommendation 5.2: The number of nurse researchers should be increased to prepare to build the knowledge base in environmental health as it relates to the practice of nursing.*

**Rationale:** Few researchers, nurse or nonnurse, have published data and findings that support environmental health in the clinical practice of nursing. Of this very small number, the researchers contributing to the knowledge base for clinical nursing practice and environmental health are almost exclusively nurses. Nurse researchers are also the faculty most likely to incorporate research findings into the curricula of nursing education programs.

### Strategies for Achieving Recommendation 5.2:

1. Increase the numbers of new investigator awards available to nurse researchers in environmental health.

2. Create mechanisms for recognizing achievement in developing the body of knowledge in environmental health.

3. Use research and other funding mechanisms to create centers of research excellence in environmental health with nurse researcher principal investigators.

4. Create incentives for faculty in general and for faculty of schools of nursing and other units of higher education to incorporate environmental health content into a research-based curriculum.

5. Plan consensus and other conferences in which nursing and other faculty can identify and coalesce current research-based content in environmental health with regard to the clinical practice of nursing.

6. Provide incentives for nursing faculty to develop expertise in environmental health.

### Priorities for Nursing Research in Environmental Health

*Recommendation 5.3: Research priorities for nursing in environmental health should be established and used by funding agencies for resource allocation decisions and to give direction to nurse researchers.*

**Rationale:** The descriptive nature of the existing nursing research in environmental health suggests an underdeveloped approach to building the knowledge base for clinical practice. In addition, despite the breadth of topical areas, nursing research in environmental health lacks depth in any one area.

### Strategies for Achieving Recommendation 5.3:

1. Use multidisciplinary teams of experts in environmental health (including nurse researchers, advanced-practice nurses, and public health nurses) jointly to identify the nursing research priorities.

2. Include private-sector corporations in setting priorities for funding.

3. Provide incentives for nurse researchers to be primary investigators on interdisciplinary research directed towards the clinical practice of nursing.

4. Encourage joint programs among different institutions to help achieve "critical mass" and to have the broadest possible impact.

### Dissemination of Research Findings

*Recommendation 5.4: Current efforts to disseminate research findings to nurses, other health care providers, and the public should be strengthened and expanded.*

**Rationale:** The impact of research on nursing practice is enhanced by effectively communicating the research findings to nurses, other health care professionals, and the public. For this reason, it is important that the findings be published in peer-reviewed journals and other media—including nursing and interdisciplinary journals as well as the public press—that will reach the appropriate target audiences. An emphasis on interdisciplinary dissemination is particularly important in regard to occupational and environmental health research.

### Strategies for Achieving Recommendation 5.4:

1. In addition to publishing reports, articles, and other documents, the dissemination of environmental health research results at a wide variety of professional meetings should also be pursued (e.g., through presentations and posters).

2. Researchers should be encouraged to share research instruments as a way of furthering the body of knowledge and the replication of studies.

3. Focused research conferences on environmental health in nursing could be used to disseminate research findings to nurse clinicians and educators.

# References

AACN (American Association of Colleges of Nursing). 1986. Essentials of College and University Education for Professional Nursing: Final Report. Washington, DC: AACN.

AACN. 1991. Nursing Education's Agenda for the 21st Century. Washington, DC: AACN.

AACN. 1994. Certification and Regulation of Advanced Practice Nurses: Position Statement. Washington, DC: AACN.

AACN. 1995. AACN 1994–1995 Enrollment and Graduations Baccalaureate and Graduate Programs in Nursing. Washington, DC: AACN.

ACHNE (Association of Community Health Nursing Educators). 1991. Essentials of Master's Nursing Education for Advanced Community Health Nursing. Lexington, KY: ACHNE.

ACHNE. 1992. Essentials of Baccalaureate Nursing Education for Entry Level Practice in Community Health Nursing. Skokie, IL: ACHNE.

Aiken, L.H. and Salmon, M.E. 1994. Health care work force priorities: What should nursing do now? Inquiry 31:318–29.

Amler, R.W., and Lybarger, J.A. 1993. Research program for neurotoxic disorders and other adverse health outcomes at hazardous chemical sites in the United States of America. Environmental Research 61(2):279–84.

ANA (American Nurses Association). 1980. A Conceptual Model of Community Health Nursing. Kansas City, MO: ANA.

ANA. 1986. Standards of Community Health Nursing Practice. Kansas City, MO: ANA.

ANA. 1991. Nursing Agenda for Health Care Reform. Washington, DC: ANA.

Anderson, E.T., and McFarlane, J.M. 1995. Community as Partner: Theory and Practice of Nursing. Philadelphia: J.B. Lippincott.

APHA (American Public Health Association). 1980. The Definition and Role of Public Health Nursing in the Delivery of Health Care: A Statement of the Public Health Nursing Section. Washington, DC: American Public Health Association.

Ashford, N.A. 1994. Monitoring the worker and the community exposure and disease: Legal and ethical considerations in the U.S. Clinical Chemistry 40(7):1426–37.

ATS (American Thoracic Society). 1990. Environmental controls and lung disease. American Review of Respiratory Disease 142:915.

ATSDR. 1988. The Nature and Extent of Lead Poisoning in Children in the U.S.: A Report to Congress. Atlanta: Department of Health and Human Services.

ATSDR. 1991. Case Studies in Environmental Medicine (No. 16)—Nitrate/Nitrite Toxicity. Atlanta: Department of Health and Human Services.

ATSDR. 1992. Case Studies in Environmental Medicine (No. 26)—Taking an Exposure History. Atlanta: Department of Health and Human Services.

Baldwin, D., Johnson, J., and Hill, P. 1994. Student satisfaction with classroom use of computer-assisted instruction. Nursing Outlook 42:188–92.

Barnes, D., Eribes, C., Juarbe, T., Nelson, M., Proctor, S., Sawyer, L., Shaul, M., and Meleis, A.I. 1995. Primary health care and primary care: A confusion of philosophies. Nursing Outlook 43(1):7–16.

Bellack, J.P., Musham, C., Hainer, A., Graber, D.R., and Holmes, D. 1995. Environmental Health Competencies: A Survey of U.S. Nurse Practitioner Programs. Unpublished Report. Charleston: Medical University of South Carolina.

BLS (Bureau of Labor Statistics). 1995. Work injuries and illnesses by selected characteristics, 1993. Washington, DC: Department of Labor News, April 26.

BLS. 1995. National Census of Fatal Occupational Injuries, 1993. Washington, DC: Department of Labor, May 15.

Boex, J.R., Gary, M., Edwards, J., Marder, W., and Politzer, R. 1993. Primary Care Practitioners: Analyses of Competencies, Costs, and Quality of Care and the Effect of Training Upon Their Supply. Ann Arbor, MI: W.K. Kellogg Foundation.

Bowers, J.J. 1994. Letter on Behalf of ANCC Certification Query for Environmental Health Nursing. Washington, DC: American Nurses Credentialing Center, September 27.

Brown, S.A., Duchin, S.P., and Villagomez, E.T. 1992. Diabetes education in a Mexican American population: pilot testing of a research videotape. Diabetes Educator 1:47–51.

Buckler, G. 1994. The effect of indoor air quality on health. Imprint 41(3):60–5, 93.

Bullough, B., and Bullough, V. 1990. Nursing in the Community. St. Louis: C.V. Mosby.

CDC (Centers for Disease Control and Prevention). 1991a. Preventing Lead Poisoning in Young Children. Atlanta: Department of Health and Human Services.

CDC. 1991b. Assessment Protocol for Excellence in Public Health. Atlanta: CDC and National Association of County Health Officials.

CDC. 1995. Deaths from Melanoma—United States, 1973–1992. Morbidity and Mortality Weekly Report, May 5.

CEPH (Council on Education for Public Health). 1986. Accreditation Criteria for Graduate Schools of Public Health. Washington, DC: CEPH.

CEPH. 1993. Accreditation Criteria for Graduate Schools of Public Health. Washington, DC: CEPH.

Chiras, D.D. 1994. Environmental Science: Action for a Sustainable Future. Redwood City, CA.: Benjamin/Cummings Publishing.

Chivian, E., McCally, M., Hu, H., and Haines, A. 1993. Critical Condition: Human Health and the Environment. Cambridge, MA: MIT Press.

Clawson, K., and Osterweis, M., eds. 1993. The Roles of Physician Assistants and Nurse Practitioners in Primary Care. Washington, DC: Association of Academic Health Centers.

Clemen-Stone, S., Eigsti, D.G., and McGuire, S.L. 1995. Comprehensive Family and Community Health Nursing. 4th ed. St. Louis: C.V. Mosby.

CPHF (California Public Health Foundation). 1992. Kids and the Environment: Toxic Hazards, A Course on Pediatric Environmental Health. Berkeley: CPHF.

Cutter, S.L. 1993. Living With Risk. New York: Routledge, Chapman, and Hall, Inc.

Davis, A.J., and Aroskar, M.A. 1991. *Ethical Dilemmas in Nursing Practice*. 3rd ed. Norwalk, CT: Appleton and Lange.

Davis, M.E.P. 1990. Construction, sanitation, and hygiene. American Journal Nursing 1(2):133.

Daynes, R.A. 1990. Immune system and ultraviolet light. In Global Atmospheric Change and Public Health, J.C. White, ed. New York: Elsevier.

DeAngelis, C.D. 1994. Nurse practitioner redux. JAMA 271(11):868–71.

Demers, P. 1990. Occupational exposure to electromagnetic radiation and breast cancer in males. American Journal of Epidemiology 132:775–6.

DeWitt, K. 1990. Specialties in nursing. American Journal of Nursing 1(1):14–17.

DHHS (Department of Health and Human Services). 1979. Healthy People 2000: The Surgeon General's Report on Health Promotion and Disease Prevention. Pub No. HRS-P-OD-90-1. Washington, DC: Government Printing Office.

DHHS. 1986. The Health Consequences of Involuntary Smoking: A Report of the Surgeon General. Pub. No. 87-8398. Washington, DC: Government Printing Office.

DHHS. 1988. Evaluating the Environmental Health Workforce. Pub. No. 0907160. Washington, DC: Health Resources and Services Administration.

DHHS. 1990. Healthy People 2000: The Surgeon General's Report on Health Promotion and Disease Prevention. Pub. No. 91-50212. Washington, DC: Government Printing Office.

DHHS. 1990. Seventh Report to the President and Congress on the Status of Health Personnel. Washington, DC: DHHS.

DHHS. 1991. Educational Resource Centers. Cincinnati, OH: Division of Training and Manpower Development, National Institute of Occupational Health.

Donaldson, S. 1995. Nursing Science for Nursing Practice (chapter 1). In Search of Nursing Science, A. Omery et al., eds. Thousand Oaks, CA: Sage Publications, Inc.

Donaldson, S., and Crowley, D. 1978. The discipline of nursing. Nursing Outlook 26(22):113–20.

Environmental Studies Board, Commission on Natural Resources. 1988. Urban Pest Management. Washington, DC: National Academy Press.

EPA (Environmental Protection Agency). 1990. Evaluation of the Potential Carcinogenicity of Electromagnetic Fields. Pub. No. EPA/600/6–9/005A. Washington, DC: EPA.

EPA. 1992. Environmental Equity: Reducing Risk for All Communities. Pub. No. EPA 230-R-92-008. Washington, DC: EPA.

Fagin, C.M., and Lynaugh, J.E. 1992. Reaping the rewards of radical change: A new agenda for nursing education. Nursing Outlook 40(5):213–20.

Gary, F., and Kavanagh, C.T. 1991. *Psychiatric Mental Health Nursing*. Philadelphia: J.B. Lippincott.

Goldman, R.H., and Peters, J.M. 1981. The occupational and environmental health history. JAMA 246(24):2831–36.

Gorall, A.H., May, L.A., and Mulley, A.G. 1995. *Primary Care Medicine*. 3rd ed. Philadelphia: J.B. Lippincott.

Gortner, S. 1990. Nursing values and science: Toward a science philosophy. Image: Journal of Nursing Scholarship 22(2):101–8.

Green, L.W. 1990. *Community Health*. 6th ed. St. Louis: Times Mirror/Mosby.

Haines, A. 1993. The possible effects of climate change on health. In Critical Condition: Human Health and the Environment, M. Chivian et al., eds. Cambridge, MA: MIT Press.

Havens, B.B., and Stevens, R. 1990. A continuing education model for community health nursing practice. Journal of Community Health Nursing 7(3):123–30.

Hersey, P. et al. 1983. Alteration in T cell subsets and induction of suppressor T cell activity in normal subjects after exposure to sunlight. Journal of Immunology 31:171–4.

HRSA (Health Resources and Services Administration). 1992. Registered Nurse Population as Findings from the Sample Survey of Registered Nurses: March 1992. Rockville, MD: Division of Nursing, HRSA.

Hu, H. 1990. Effects of ultraviolet radiation. Medical Clinics of North America 74:509–14.

ICN (International Council of Nurses). 1986. The Nurse's Role in Safeguarding the Human Environment. Geneva, Switzerland: International Council of Nurses.

INFORM, Inc. 1995. Toxics Watch 1995. New York: INFORM, Inc.

IOM (Institute of Medicine). 1988. Future of Public Health. Washington, DC: National Academy Press.

IOM. 1993. Indoor Allergins: Assessing and Controlling Adverse Health Effects. Washington, DC: National Academy Press.

IOM. 1995. Environmental Medicine: Integrating a Missing Element into Medical Education. Washington, DC: National Academy Press.

Jacques, P.F., and Chylack, L.T., Jr. 1991. Epidemiologic evidence of a role for the antioxidant vitamins and carotenoids in cataract prevention. American Journal of Clinical Nutrition 53 (Suppl. 1): 352S–5S.

Jones, D.C., Davis, J.A., and Davis, M.C. 1987. Public Health Nursing Education and Practice. Springfield, VA: Department of Health and Human Services.

Kalisch, P.A., and Kalisch, B.J. 1986. The Advance of Nursing, 2nd ed. Boston: Little, Brown and Co.

Keatinge, W.R., Coleshaw, S.R., and Eastern, J.C. 1986. Increased platelet and red cell counts, blood viscosity and plasma cholesterol levels during heat stress and mortality from coronary and cerebral thrombosis. American Journal of Medicine 81:795–800.

Kilbourne, EM. 1990. Heat waves: The Public Health Consequences of Disasters. Atlanta: Department of Health and Human Services.

Koch, E.W., Rankin, J.A., and Stewart, R. 1990. Nursing students' preferences in the use of computer assisted learning. Journal of Nursing Education 29:122–6.

Langford, T.L. 1990. Rural health care in the 'future perfect.' Academic Medicine 65(suppl 12):540–542.

Leikauf, G.D. 1992. Formaldehyde and other aldehydes. In Environmental Toxicants: Human Exposures and Their Health Effects, M. Lippmann, ed. New York: Van Nostrand Reinhold.

Lindberg, J.B., Hunter, M.L., and Kruszewski, A.Z. 1994. Introduction to Nursing: Concepts, Issues and Opportunities. 2nd ed. Philadelphia: J.B. Lippincott.

Lindeman, C. 1993. President's message: To prepare a preventionist. Nursing and Health Care 14(9):486.

Lipscomb, J. 1994a. Environmental Health Curricula. Presentation at the Institute of Medicine, Committee on Enhancing Environmental Health Content in the Practice of Nursing, Washington, DC, August 4.

Lipscomb, J. 1994b. Environmental health: Assuming a leadership role. AAOHN Journal 42(7):314–5.

Longstreth, J. 1990. Skin cancer and ultraviolet light: Risk estimates due to ozone depletion. In Global Atmospheric Change and Public Health, J.C. White, ed. New York: Elsevier.

Lowdermilk, D.L., and Fishel, A.H. 1991. Computer simulations as a measure of nursing students' decision-making skills. Journal of Nursing Education 30(1):34–9.

Lybarger, J.A., Spengler, R.F., and DeRosa, C.T. 1993. Priority Health Conditions: An Integrated Strategy to Evaluate the Relationship Between Illness and Exposure to Hazardous Substances. Atlanta: Agency for Toxic Substances and Disease Registry.

Lynaugh, J.E., and Fagin, C.M. 1988. Nursing comes of age. Image: Journal of Nursing Scholarship 20(4):184–90.

Marquis, B.L., and Huston, C.J. 1992. *Leadership Roles and Management Functions in Nursing.* Philadelphia: J.B. Lippincott.

Maston, Y., and Connover, K.P. 1990. Automated continuing education and patient education. Computers in Nursing 8(4):144–50.

Matanowski, G., Elliot, F., and Breysse, P. 1989. Cancer Incidence in New York Telephone Workers. New York: Electric Power Research Institute.

Mausner, J.S., and Kramer, S. 1985. Epidemiology: An Introductory Text. Philadelphia: W.B. Saunders.

McLaughlin, F.E., and Marasuilo, L.A. 1990. *Advanced Nursing and Health Care Research.* Philadelphia: W.B. Saunders.

Miller, T. 1993. Environmental Science: Sustaining the Earth, 4th ed. Belmont, CA: Wadsworth Publishing Co.

Moore, E.J. 1990. Visiting nurse. American Journal of Nursing 1(1):17–21.

Morrow, M.M. 1992. Medicare Physician Payment Reform: Implications for Nurse Practitioners. Journal of the American Academy of Nurse Practitioners 4(1):38–43.

Moses, M. 1993. Pesticides. In Occupational and Environmental Reproductive Hazards, M. Paul, ed. Baltimore, MD: Williams and Wilkens.

Mundinger, M.O. 1994. Advanced-practice nursing—good medicine for physicians? New England Journal of Medicine 330(3):211–4.

Murray, R.B., and Zentner, J.P. 1989. *Nursing Assessment and Health Promotion: Strategies Through the Life Span.* 4th ed. Norwalk, CT: Appleton & Lange.

NACHO (National Association of County Health Officials). 1991. APEX—Public Health. Washington, DC: NACHO and Centers for Disease Control and Prevention.

Narkunas, D., Hibbs, B., Phillips, L., Middleton, D., and Lum, M. 1994. Clues to Unraveling the Association Between Illness and Environmental Exposure. Atlanta: Agency for Toxic Substances and Disease Registry.

NCSBN (National Council of State Boards of Nursing). 1994. Profiles of Member Boards— 1994. Chicago, NCSBN.

NCNR (National Center for Nursing Research). 1993. National Nursing Research Agenda: Developing Knowledge for Practice: Challenges and Opportunities. Bethesda, MD: NCNR.

Needleman, H.L., Gunnoe, C., Leviton, A., Reed, R., Peresie, H., Maher, C., and Barrett, P. 1979. Deficits in psychologic and classroom performance of children with elevated dentine lead levels. New England Journal of Medicine 300(13):689–95.

Needleman, H.L., and Landrigan, P.J. 1994. Raising Children Toxic Free. New York: Farrar, Straus & Giroux, Inc.

Needleman, H.L., Schell, A., Bellinger, D., Leviton, A., and Allred, E.N. 1990. The long-term effects of exposure to low doses of lead in childhood: An 11-year follow-up report. New England Journal of Medicine 322(2):83–8.

Neufer, L. 1994. The role of the community health nurses in environmental health. Public Health Nursing 11(3):155–62.

Nightingale, F. 1860. Notes on Nursing: What It Is and What It Is Not. New York: D. Appleton and Co. Reprint, 1969. New York: Dover Publications, Inc.

NLN (National League for Nursing). 1992. An Agenda for Nursing Education Reform in Support of Nursing—Agenda for Health Care Reform. New York: NLN.

NLN. 1994. Nursing Data Review—1994. New York: NLN.

NRC (National Research Council). 1984. Toxicity Testing: Strategies to Determine Needs and Priorities. Washington, DC: National Academy Press.

NRC. 1986. Environmental Tobacco Smoke: Measuring Exposures and Assessing Health Effects. Washington, DC: National Academy Press.

NRC. 1991. Environmental Epidemiology: Public Health and Hazardous Wastes. Washington, DC: National Academy Press.

NRC. 1993a. Understanding and Preventing Violence. Washington, DC: National Academy Press.

NRC. 1993b. Pesticides in the Diets of Infants and Children. Washington, DC: National Academy Press.

O'Reilly, MB. 1990. Work for nurses in play-schools. American Journal of Nursing 1(1):37–9.

Oermann, M.H. 1994. Professional nursing education in the future: Changes and challenges. JOGNN 23(2):153–9.

Ostwalt, S., and Josten, L. 1994. Preparation of Public Health Nurses for Leadership Positions. Presentation at the Association of Community Health Nursing Educators Conference, San Antonio, Texas, June.

Paul, M. 1993. Occupational and Environmental Reproductive Hazards: A Guide for Clinicians. Baltimore, MD: Williams & Wilkins.

Paul, R.W. 1993. Critical Thinking: How to Prepare Students for a Rapidly Changing World. Santa Rosa, CA: Foundation for Critical Thinking.

Pender, N.J. 1992. Environmental compatibility: accepting the challenge. Nursing Outlook 40(5):200–1.

PHS (Public Health Service). 1992. Nursing: Eighth Report to the President and Congress on the Status of Health Personnel. Washington, DC: PHS.

PHS. 1994. Public Health in America. Washington, DC: PHS.

Pierson, M.H. 1990. The Orange visiting nurses' settlement. American Journal of Nursing 1(4):276–7.

Polit, D.F., and Hungler, B.P. 1995. Nursing Research: Principles and Methods. 5th ed. Philadelphia: J.B. Lippincott.

Prescott, P. 1993. Nursing: An important component of hospital survival under a reformed health care system. Nursing Economics 11(4).

Redman, B. 1994. Nursing Practice in the Changing Environment of Health Care Reform. Presentation to the IOM Committee on Enhancing Environmental Health Content in Nursing Practice, August 4, 1994; Washington, DC.

Rogers, B. 1991. Occupational health nursing education: Curricular content in baccalaureate programs. AAOHN Journal 39(3):101–8.

Rogers, B. 1994. Linkage in environmental and occupational health: Assessing, detecting, and containing exposure sources. AAOHN Journal 42(7):336–43.

Rom, W.N., ed. 1992. Environmental and Occupational Medicine, 2nd ed. Boston: Little, Brown and Co.

Rosenthal, F.S., Bakalian, A.E., Lou, C.Q., and Taylor, H.R. 1988. The effects of sunglasses on ocular exposure to ultraviolet radiation. American Journal of Public Health 78(1):72–4.

Rutstein, D.D., Mullan, R.J., Frazier, T.M., Halperin, W.E., Melius, J.M, and Sestito, J.P. 1983. Sentinel health events (occupational): A basis for physician recognition and public health surveillance. American Journal of Public Health 73(9):1054–62.

Safriet, B.J. 1994. Health care dollars and regulatory sense. Yale Journal of Regulation 9(2):15–20.

Samet, J.M., Marbury, M.C., and Spengler, J.D. 1987. Health effects and sources of indoor air pollution. Part I. American Review of Respiratory Disease 136:1486–90.

Saucier, K.A. 1991. Perspectives on Family and Community Health. St. Louis: C.V. Mosby.

Savitz, D.A. 1988. Case-control study of childhood cancers and exposure to 60 Hz magnetic fields: Review of epidemiological surveys. American Journal of Epidemiology 128(1):21–38.

Savitz, D.A., and Loomis, D.P. 1995. Magnetic field exposure in relation to leukemia and brain cancer mortality among electric utility workers. American Journal of Epidemiology 141(2):123–34.

Schare, B.L., Dunn, S.C., Clark, H.M., Soled, S.W., and Gilman, B.G. 1991. The effects of interactive video on cognitive achievement and attitude toward learning. Journal of Nursing Education 30(3):109–13.

Schulte, P.A. 1988. The role of genetic factors in bladder cancer. 1988. Cancer Detection and Prevention 11:379–88.

Schuster, E.A., and Brown, C.L., eds. 1994. Exploring Our Environmental Connections. New York: National League for Nursing Press.

Scovil, E.R. 1990. Openings for nurses. American Journal of Nursing 1(6):439–43.

Selby, M.L., Riportella-Muller, R., Quade, D., Legault, C., and Salmon, M.E. 1990. Core curriculum for master's-level community health nursing education: A comparison of the views of leaders in service and education. Public Health Nursing 7(3):150–60.

Sherman, J. 1988. Chemical Exposure and Disease. New York: Van Nostrand Reinhold.

Shugars, D.A., O'Neal, E.H., and Bader, J.D., eds. 1991a. Healthy America: Practitioners for 2005, An Agenda for Action for U.S. Health Professions Schools. Durham, NC: The Pew Health Professions Commission.

Shugars, D.A., O'Neil, E.H., and Bader, J.D. 1991b. Survey of Practitioners' Perceptions of Their Education. Durham, NC: The Pew Health Professions Commission.

Snyder, M.A., Ruth, M.V., Sattler, B., and Strasser, J. 1994. Environmental and occupational health education: A survey of community health nurses' need for educational programs. AAOHN Journal 42(7):325–8.

SCCEN (Southern Council on Collegiate Education for Nursing). 1994. Strategies for Graduate Faculty Internal Demands Versus External Realities. Atlanta: SCCEN.

Stanhope, M., and Lancaster, J. 1992. Community Health Nursing: Process and Practice for Promoting Health. 3rd ed. St. Louis: C.V. Mosby.

Stevens, P., and Hall, J. 1993. Environmental health. In Swanson, J. and Albracht, M. eds., Community Health Nursing, J. Swanson and M. Albracht, eds. Philadelphia: W.B. Saunders.

Suro, R. 1992. Rash of Birth Defects in New Borns Disturbs Border City in Texas. New York Times 31 May:3.

Tarcher, A.B., ed. 1992. Principles and Practice of Environmental Medicine. New York: Plenum Publishing Co.

Taylor, H.R. 1990. Cataracts and ultraviolet light. In Global Atmospheric Changes and Public Health, J.C. White, ed. New York: Elsevier.

Topf, M. 1994. Theoretical considerations for research on environmental stress and health. Image: Journal of Nursing Scholarship 26(4):289–93.

Waltz, C., Strickland, O.L., and Lenz, E. 1991. Measurement in Nursing Research. 2nd ed. Philadelphia: F.A. Davis.

Wertheimer, N., and Leeper, E. 1986. Possible effects of electric blankets and heated waterbeds on fetal development. Bioelectromagnetics 7(1):13–22.

Wertheimer, N., and Leeper, E. 1989. Fetal loss associated with two seasonal sources of electromagnetic field exposures. American Journal of Epidemiology 129:220–4.

Wold, S.J. 1990. Community Health Nursing: Issues and Topics. Norwalk, CT: Appleton and Lange.

World Health Organization. 1978. Primary Health Care: Report of the International Conference on Primary Health Care. Geneva: WHO.

Yunginger, J.W., Reed, C.E., O'Connell, E.J., Melton, L.J., O'Fallon, W.M., and Silverstein, M.D. 1992. A community-based study of the epidemiology of asthma. American Review of Respiratory Disease 146(4):888–94.

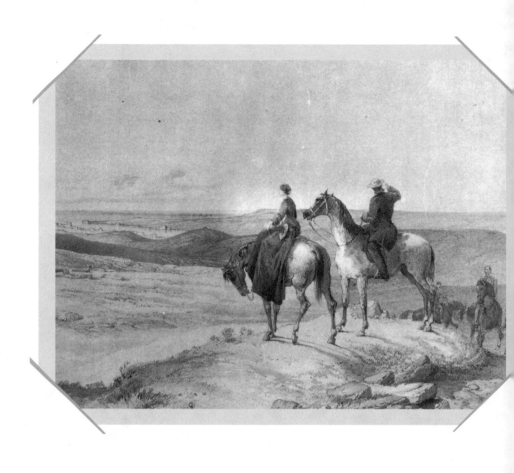

*Florence Nightingale on horseback with her friends (Mr. Bracebridge
and others) on Cathcart's Heights near Sebastopol, May 1855.*

*Sketched on the spot by her friend Selina Mills, afterward Lady Bracebridge.
Lithograph made from the finished drawing by Lady Verney and Lady Anne Blunt.
Privately issued.
Property of Duke University Medical Center Library,
History of Medicine Collections, Durham, NC.*

# Appendixes

# A
# Position Statement from the International Council of Nurses: The Nurse's Role in Safeguarding the Human Environment[*]

The preservation and improvement of the human environment has become increasingly important for man's survival and well-being. The vastness and urgency of the task place on every individual and every professional group the responsibility to participate in the efforts to safeguard man's environment, to conserve the world's resources, to study how their use affects man, and how adverse effects can be avoided.

THE NURSE'S ROLE IS TO:

Help detect ill effects of the environment on the health of man, and vice-versa. The nurse should:

- apply observational skills for the detection of ill effects of environment on the individual;
- observe individuals in all settings for effects of pollutants in order to advise on protective and/or curative measures;
- record and analyze observations made of ill effects on environment and/or pollutants on individuals;

---

*From International Council of Nurses, *The Nurse's Role in Safeguarding the Human Environment*. Position Statement. 1986. Geneva, Switzerland. Used with permission of the International Council of Nurses.

• be informed and report observations of the ecological consequences of pollutants and their adverse effects on the human being.

Be informed and apply knowledge in daily work with individuals, families, and/or community groups as to the data available on potential health hazards and ways to prevent and/or reduce them. The nurse should be informed about:

• the studies and identification of the environmental problems at local, national, and international level;
• their effects on man;
• the standards for the protection of the human organism, especially from pollutants;
• ways to prevent and/or reduce health hazards.

Be informed and teach preventive measures about health hazards due to environmental factors as well as about conservation of environmental resources to the individual, families, and/or community groups. The nurse can:

• request and attend continuing education programs about the study of the environment and the application of this knowledge in daily life and work;
• provide health education for both the general public and health personnel in order to create awareness of environmental issues and to involve the public with environmental management and control;
• apply knowledge in areas where nursing intervention may prevent or reduce health hazards;
• report on steps taken to control the significant environmental problems of the area.

Work with health authorities in pointing out health care aspects and health hazards in existing human settlements and in the planning of new settlements. Nurses can:

• participate in exchange of information and experience about similar environmental problems with authorities in other areas;
• cooperate with health authorities in the preparation of programs to enable national and local authorities to influence their own environments;
• participate in the promotion of legislation to improve health care and reduce/prevent health hazards, and encourage the enforcement of such legislation where/when appropriate;

- participate in national/local pre-disaster planning; and cooperate in international programs in case of disasters in other countries.

Assist communities in their action on environmental health problems. The nurse can assist communities in programs to:

- reduce harmful pollutants (chemical, biological or physical, e.g., noise) in air, soil, water, and food by industries or other human efforts;
- improve nutrition;
- encourage family planning;
- assess environmental factors in work situations and pursue activities for the elimination or reduction of hazards;
- educate the general public and all levels of nursing personnel in environmental and other health hazards, especially those related to unacceptable levels of contamination.

Participate in research providing data for early warning and prevention of deleterious effects of the various environmental agents to which man is increasingly exposed; and research conducive to discovering ways and means of improving living and working conditions. The nurse, as principal investigator or in collaboration with other nurses or related professions, can carry out epidemiological and experimental research designed to provide data for:

- early warning for prevention of health hazards;
- improving living and working conditions;
- monitoring the environmental levels of pollutants;
- measuring the impact of nursing intervention on environmental hazards.

# B

# Environmental Hazards for the Nurse as a Worker[*]

Nursing is a uniquely hazardous occupation. This appendix summarizes some of the major hazards nurses may face on-the-job, and provides statistics for illnesses and injuries among nurses associated with working conditions. This discussion will illustrate the pervasive nature of environmental and occupational hazards in a setting familiar to the reader.

The Bureau of Labor Statistics reports that there are 1,859,000 RNs (1993) and 659,000 LPNs (1992) employed in the United States. Of the 2,518,000 nurses, 882,647 (35%) are employed in hospitals, and the rest in other health care settings including but not limited to nursing homes, health maintenance organizations, physicians' offices, community health agencies, schools, and corporations.

In 1992, the rate of occupational injury and illness for nurses in health care settings was 18.6% per 100 full-time workers (18.2% accounted for injuries). This is higher than for hazardous occupations such as heavy construction where the rate of occupational injury and illness is 13.8% per 100 full-time workers or mining where the total is 7.5% per 100 full-time workers (DiBenedetto, 1995).

---

[*]Appendix B, *Environmental Hazards for the Nurse as a Worker*, was written by committee member Gail F. Buckler. Ms. Buckler is a clinical instructor in the Environmental and Occupational Health Sciences Institute, University of Medicine and Dentistry of New Jersey-Robert Wood Johnson Medical School and Rutgers, the State University of New Jersey, and assistant professor of clinical nursing, School of Nursing, UMDNJ.

Nurses confront potential exposure to infectious diseases, toxic substances, back injuries, and radiation. They also are subject to hazards such as stress, shift work, and violence in the workplace. These typically fall under the broad categories of chemical, biological, physical, and psychosocial hazards.

## INFECTIOUS DISEASES

The risk of infections is present not only in hospitals but in other settings where nurses are employed such as nursing homes, institutions for the retarded, prisons, and outpatient facilities, i.e.: dialysis centers, workplace health centers, or community health clinics. In hospitals high risk areas include pediatric areas, infectious disease wards, emergency rooms, and ambulatory care facilities.

Hepatitis B (HBV) is the most prevalent work-related infectious disease in the United States. Although blood is the major source of the virus, it may also be present in saliva, semen, and feces. Transmission may occur from a percutaneous stick from a contaminated needle or other sharp instrument (the risk of contracting HBV after a stick with a known contaminated needle is 6–30 percent) (Udasin and Gochfeld, 1994), after contaminated blood enters a break in the skin or splatters onto mucous membranes, or upon ingestion. The OSHA Bloodborne Pathogens Standard has provisions for preventing Hepatitis B in healthcare workers including Hepatitis B vaccine, education, procedures for sterilization and disinfection, and use of personal protective clothing. In addition, the CDC has recommendations for work practices during invasive procedures.

Hepatitis A poses a risk for workers in settings such as institutions for the retarded where personal hygiene may be poor (Levy and Wegman, 1995). The use of good handwashing techniques is the most effective preventive measure for this virus.

Delta hepatitis occurs only in patients who are infected with Hepatitis B (Levy and Wegman, 1995). This occurs mainly in IV drug abusers, and hemophiliacs and may be transmitted to patients who undergo hemodialysis. The preventive measures utilized to minimize the spread of Hepatitis B should be instituted to limit the transmission of Delta hepatitis.

The majority of cases of Hepatitis C are associated with IV drug use or are idiopathic in origin. The disease has rarely been transmitted to health care personnel via percutaneous exposure. Additional research is needed to determine the extent of this disease as an occupational hazard.

The United States experienced a resurgence of tuberculosis in the 1990s. This is attributed to the HIV epidemic, an increase in immigration from Asia, homelessness, and the emergence of drug-resistant strains of tuberculosis. Nurses employed in hospitals (particularly in emergency departments, pulmonary departments, and HIV units), long term care facilities, outpatient clinics and prisons are at risk for contracting tuberculosis (Hellman and Gram, 1993; Levy and Wegman, 1995). Often the patients who they come in contact with are undiagnosed (Hellman and Gram, 1993). The CDC has recommendations for tuberculosis infection control and OSHA will be issuing its proposed tuberculosis standard in the near future.

Nurses in many settings may be exposed to infectious diseases such as measles, mumps, rubella, and influenza. Immune status should be determined when feasible for employees with direct patient care responsibilities and appropriate immunizations should be offered.

Human immunodeficiency virus may be acquired by exposure to infected blood or body fluids. The risk of contracting HIV after percutaneous exposure with a contaminated needle is 0.3–0.4 percent (Udasin and Gochfeld, 1994). Of the 42 documented seroconversions in health care workers, 13 were nurses (HIV/AIDS Surveillance Report—CDC). The OSHA Bloodborne Pathogens Standard's published guidelines are designed to prevent occupational exposure to HIV. The CDC recommends that blood and body fluids of all patients be considered potentially infectious and, consequently, universal precautions should be adhered to with each patient contact.

## TOXIC EXPOSURES

Antineoplastic agents may be prepared and administered in a variety of clinical settings. A number of studies have documented the hazards of cytotoxic drugs to nurses who work with them. These agents have been associated with mutagenic, teratogenic, and carcinogenic effects as well as adverse effects such as irritation of the skin, eyes, and mucous membranes or acute allergic reactions (Rogers, 1987). Improper handling, i.e., mixing of these agents contribute to exposure in workers. OSHA guidelines and recommendations by several professional associations exist for safe handling of antineoplastic agents.

Ethylene oxide is commonly used in hospitals to sterilize medical instruments and heat-sensitive substances and may be encountered in central supply, surgical services, and patient care areas. It is documented that this agent possesses carcinogenic, mutagenic, and teratogenic properties. It is also associated with respiratory tract irritation, central nervous system effects, and chemical burns (U.S. Department of Health and Human Services, 1988). OSHA has a standard designed to protect workers from exposure to ethylene oxide.

Exposure to waste anesthetic gases may occur in operating rooms, labor and delivery, and recovery rooms. Long-term exposure to these agents have been associated with an increased risk of renal (methoxyflurane) and hepatic (halothane) disorders and have also been correlated with an increased risk of spontaneous abortions and congenital abnormalities (nitrous oxide) in exposed workers. There are no standards published by OSHA for waste anesthetic gases, however, the National Institute for Occupational Safety and Health (NIOSH) has recommended exposure limits for nitrous oxide and the halogenated compounds.

Nurses have potential exposure to formaldehyde when they work in renal dialysis units, during the transfer of tissue to formalin in preparation for pathology, and as a residue when it is used for the disinfection of operating rooms. Formaldehyde is associated with irritant and allergic dermatitis, eye irritation, and occupational asthma. It is considered a possible human carcinogen. OSHA has a standard which limits worker exposure to formaldehyde.

Glutaraldehye is a germicide used in the cold sterilization of instruments. Nurses who perform cold sterilization in dialysis, endoscopy, and intensive care units are subject to exposure. Exposure has been linked to the practice of soaking instruments in open containers without benefit of local exhaust ventilation as well as during manual cleaning of instruments. It is a skin and mucous membrane irritant. It may also cause skin sensitization, asthma-like symptoms, headache, and flu-like symptoms. At high levels of exposure, it has been associated with liver toxicity. OSHA has determined that symptoms may be induced by airborne concentrations of 0.3 ppm or greater. A NIOSH study showed that routine use of glutaraldehyde in hospitals produced personal breathing zone and ambient air levels of 0.4 ppm (Wiggins et al., 1989). A ceiling limit (maximum allowable level at any time) of 0.2 ppm has been set by OSHA for exposure to glutaraldehyde. Reduction of exposure should take place by the use of engineering controls and good work practices.

Elemental mercury is used in various instruments found in healthcare settings. The greatest opportunity for exposure exists when there is breakage of the glass part of a thermometer or sphygmomanometer and the mercury spills onto the floor or countertop. Exposure to high levels can cause acute poisoning and death. Short term high exposures can cause pulmonary and central nervous system damage. Workers can bring mercury home on their shoes and clothing and, as a result, expose family members (Hudson et al., 1987). Prevention of toxicity can be accomplished by employee education, environmental controls, and proper handling of spills.

## BACK INJURIES

Back injury ranks second among all causes of occupational injuries for all occupations. It is reported that 40,000 nurses report back related injuries annually (Garrett et al., 1992). Nursing activities such as lifting patients in bed, helping patients out of bed, transferring patients from the bed, and carrying equipment weighing 30 pounds or greater are the most frequent causes of back pain.

Back injuries in hospital nursing personnel account for greater than half the total compensation payments for back injury and it is estimated that greater than 764,000 lost work days are incurred each year (Garrett et al., 1992). The activities performed by nursing personnel at extended care facilities place them at greater risk for back injuries. Frequent lifts and assists for patients who tend to be weak, debilitated, and elderly increase the risk of back injuries in those who provide their care. Registered nurses, licensed practical nurses, and nurse's aides are among the health care workers most frequently affected by this type of injury.

A study of workers' compensation data indicated that nurse's aides ranked fifth and LPNs ninth among all occupations in filing for work-related back injury (Fuortes et al., 1994). The incidence of low back injuries in nurse's aides was found to be at least three times greater than for nurses. Studies have revealed that newly qualified nurses or trainees are at greater risk for back injury than more experienced personnel. Additional risk factors for back injury are gender (females have higher incidence), shift (evening shift is highest risk), and weight of the nurse (excess weight and poor muscle tone influence development of lumbar lordosis and elevated intra-vertebral disc pressure).

The ergonomics of various nursing functions should be taken into consideration when developing a back injury prevention program. Protocols should be developed which take into account assessment and adjustment of specific tasks, as well as for identifying the need for assistance and type required. Training and orientation regarding lifting techniques upon initial hire and upon reassignment would be a useful preventive measure.

## RADIATION

Exposure to ionizing radiation is associated with mutagenic and teratogenic properties leading to an increased risk of miscarriage, stillbirth, and other adverse reproductive outcomes, as well as cancers such as myelogenous leukemia, bone, and skin cancer.

Nurses have potential exposure to ionizing radiation while holding patients who are undergoing radiographs, and during direct care of patients undergoing nuclear medicine tests and implants (McAbee et al., 1993). Personnel in departments where portable x-rays are performed (i.e., emergency room, surgical areas, intensive care units) are often inadvertently exposed to radiation. Although researchers differ over quantifying the amount of radiation that is hazardous, there is evidence that low levels can cause biological damage.

OSHA's standard for ionizing radiation is designed to protect workers who are not covered under the Nuclear Regulatory Commission and the exposure limit is set at three rem per quarter (of a year). The Joint Commission on Accreditation of Health Care Organizations mandates that hospitals with radiology equipment have a health physicist on staff (U.S. Department of Health and Human Services, 1988).

## STRESS

Nurses who work with terminally and chronically ill patients, and nurses who work in the intensive care units, emergency room, burn unit, or operating room are at particular risk for stress related symptoms. The early signs of stress include irritibility, loss of appetite, ulcers, migraine headaches, emotional instability, and sleep disturbances (Lewy, 1991).

Workplace factors that may contribute to stress include dealing with life-threatening illnesses and injuries, demanding patients, overwork, understaffing, difficult schedules (i.e., rotating shifts or working multiple shifts), specialized equipment, the hierarchy of authority, lack of control and participation in planning and decision making, and patient deaths. In many hospitals, the nurse may feel isolated, fatigued, angry, and powerless due to a sense of depersonalization created by a large bureaucratic system.

When the signs of stress are not recognized and treated, burnout may result. Stress-related symptoms can lead to an increase in the use of cigarettes, alcohol, and drugs. The worker's attitude and behavior may be adversely affected, leading to decreased job performance, and increased absenteeism.

Methods for coping with stress include regularly scheduled staff meetings; development of a stress management program and adequate coping mechanisms; availability of an employee assistance program; flexibility and worker participation in development of work schedules; appropriate training and educational sessions; creation of an organized and efficient work environment (to the extent that this can be accomplished); recognition and proper action on legitimate complaints; and group therapy/support groups for staff who deal with difficult professional problems.

## VIOLENCE

Nurses in mental health facilities have, for a long time, been the subjects of patient violence. Other high risk settings include emergency departments, pediatric units, medical-surgical units, and long term care facilities (Lipscomb and Love, 1992). Weapon carrying is not uncommon in psychiatric and general medical emergency rooms.

The environmental risk factors associated with assault of health care workers are inadequate training, staffing patterns, time of day, and containment practices. Studies show that inexperienced workers and nursing students are at increased risk of assault. The majority of the injuries are sustained in the process of containing patient violence and the rest are battery injuries.

Preventive measures include adequate security in high risk areas, staff training upon hire and annually, written procedures for controlling violent patients, worker participation on the hospital health and safety committee, and use of legal action against the assaultive party and the institution.

## CONCLUSION

In summary, nurses are subject to exposure to environmental hazards through their contact with patients, physical and psychological job demands, and as a result of the drugs and technology with which they work. Consequently, they have intrinsic knowledge about a variety of environmental factors that can be encountered professionally. Their enhanced understanding of these problems can be useful in accessing the environmental issues that may be faced by their patients.

## REFERENCES

Bureau of Labor Statistics, Personal Communication.

Centers for Disease Control and Prevention, HIV/AIDS Surveillance Report, 6:1, p 11.

DiBenedetto, D., Occupational Hazards of the Health Care Industry: Protecting Health Care Workers. AAOHN Journal, 1995, 43:3, pp 131–137.

Fuortes, L.J., Shi, Y., Zhang, M., et al., Epidemiology of back injury in university hospital nurses from review of workers' compensation records and a case-control survey. Journal of Occupational Medicine, 1994, 36:9, pp 1022–1031.

Garrett, B., Singiser, D., Banks, S., Back injuries among nursing personnel: the relationship of personal characteristics, risk factors, and nursing practices. AAOHN Journal, 1992, 40:11, pp 510–516.

Hellman, S.L., Gram, M.C., The resurgence of tuberculosis: risk in health care settings. AAOHN Journal, 1993, 41:2, pp 66–72.

Hudson, P., Vogt, R., et al. Elemental mercury exposure among children of thermometer plant workers. Pediatrics, 1987, 79:6, pp 935–938

Levy, B.S., Wegman, D.H., eds., *Occupational Health: Recognizing and Preventing Work-Related Disease.* Third Edition, 1995, Little, Brown and Company, pp 355–379.

Lewy, R.M., *Employees at Risk: Protecting the Health of the Health Care Worker.* 1991, Van Nostrand Reinhold, pp 112–126.

Lipscomb, J.A., Love, C.C., Violence toward health care workers: an emerging occupational hazard. AAOHN Journal, 1992, 40:5, pp 219–228.

McAbee, R.R., Galluci, B.J., Checkoway, H., Adverse reproductive outcomes and occupational exposures among nurses: an investigation of multiple hazardous exposures. AAOHN Journal, 1993, 41:3, pp 110–119.

Rogers, B., Health hazards to personnel handling antineoplastic agents. In State of the Art Reviews: Occupational Medicine, Health Problems of Health Care Workers, Emmett, E., editor, 1987, 2:3, pp 513–524.

Udasin, I., Gochfeld, M. Implications of the occupational safety and health administration's bloodborne pathogen standard for the occupational health professional, JOM, 1994, 6:5, p 549.

U.S. Department of Health and Human Services, PHS, CDC, NIOSH, *Guidelines for Protecting the Safety and Health of Health Care Workers.* 1988.

Wiggins, P., McCurdy, S., Zeidenberg, W., Epistaxis due to glutaraldehyde exposure. JOM, 1989; 31:10, pp 854–856.

# C

# Environmental Health Curricula*

The purpose of this appendix is to provide guidance on the development of environmental health curricula by defining essential curricular content, competencies, and learning objectives in environmental health as they relate to existing specialty areas and educational levels. Before doing so, however, two caveats should be kept in mind when reviewing the proposed content.

First, if nurses are truly going to make a significant contribution in the area of environmental health, they will need to develop, at a minimum, an awareness, and, ideally, some expertise in the range of areas included in the specialty area of environmental and occupational health. This is particularly true for frontline health care professionals who may be the first and sometimes only contact with members of the public who have many informational needs regarding environmental hazards. As a result, the proposed essential curricular content is comprehensive and may appear to be resource intensive upon first review. However, if it is integrated successfully, the suggested content will not be burdensome but will result in an improved overall basic nursing education, one which will better prepare nurses for future practice within the context of health care reform.

---

*This Appendix was prepared by Jane Lipscomb, R.N., Ph.D., and was presented by her to the Committee on Enhancing Environmental Health Content in Nursing Practice at the committee's second meeting on August 4, 1994.

Second, the current focus of this Institute of Medicine (IOM) initiative is environmental health. Although the committee's definition of environmental health encompasses occupational health, the two areas are not treated in parallel within this initiative, as in the 1988 IOM report on primary care physicians. This appendix is based on the committee's working definition of environmental health in its general approach to the curriculum. However, some of the content in the proposed curriculum is considered parallel between occupational health and environmental health, such as history taking and the regulatory framework.

By way of introducing the recommendations for the specific content, a nursing curriculum that incorporates essential content in environmental health must be grounded in the basic principles of epidemiology and toxicology and must incorporate the concept of risk and its application to groups and individuals. Such curricula should be viewed not only as enhancing the environmental health content of the curriculum but also as preparing nurses to more successfully contribute to overall disease prevention and health promotion efforts.

## ESSENTIAL CURRICULAR CONTENT

The essential curricular content can be grouped into the following four areas: nursing and the environment, legislation and regulations, exposure recognition and principles of control, and health consequences. The area of nursing and the environment includes a definition and framework for *environment* different from the current use of the term in nursing. This area also includes an articulation of nursing's role in promoting environmental health, for example, in areas of environmental justice and advocacy. The important area of risk perception and risk communication is also included within this category, although this content would be sequenced differently in an actual curriculum. Legislation and regulations must include an overview of major environmental and occupational legislation. Exposure assessment includes an understanding of the basic principles of toxicology, such as routes of exposure and dose (i.e., dose-response and time-dose characteristics). A basic understanding of the principles of controlling exposures is also included because this knowledge is essential to preventing environmental illnesses. Lastly, the area of health consequences includes the ability to take an environmental and occupational history, basic knowledge of sentinel environmental illnesses, and the ability to recognize when referral to a specialist is indicated.

The length of the program of study (e.g., Bachelor of Science in Nursing [BSN] versus Associate Degree [AD]) and the presence of community health- and policy-focused course work will dictate the level of detail possible. It should be the goal of all basic nursing programs to incorporate some level of each of the essential content areas into their curricula through formal didactic course work, field experiences, and/or self-study. More specific recommendations for content in these four areas follow.

1. Nursing and the Environment

— Definition of the environment (e.g., physical, chemical, and biological agents in air, food, water, and/or soil).
— Impact of the environment on the public's health and the epidemiology of major environmental illnesses.
— Role of nursing practice in promoting environment health.
— Role of advocacy in environmental health and environmental justice.
— Principles of risk perception and risk communication.

2. Legislation and Regulation

— An overview of major environmental and occupational health legislation and regulatory agencies (e.g., Environmental Protection Agency [EPA], Toxic Substances Control Act [TSCA], National Institute of Environmental Health Sciences [NIEHS], Agency of Toxic Substances and Disease Registry [ATSDR], Occupational Safety and Health Administration [OSHA], and National Institute for Occupational Safety and Health [NIOSH]).
— Environmental health resources at the national, state, and local levels.

3. Exposure Assessment

— Definitions and basic principles of hazard, exposure, and dose.
— Principle of dose-response relationship and time-dose characteristics.
— Routes of exposure to environmental contaminants.
— Process of hazard recognition and control (e.g., hierarchy of controls).

4. Health Consequences

— Environmental and occupational health screening history.
— Criteria for the work or environmental relatedness of a disease or condition.
— Indications for more in-depth history taking.
— Indications for a referral to specialists.
— Basic knowledge of environmental sentinel health events and most prevalent conditions (e.g., lead exposure or poisoning, pesticide poison-

ing, asbestos-related disease, environmentally induced or exacerbated asthma).

The competencies and learning objectives related to this content are described in the following section. A discussion of where and how to integrate this content into existing curricula is presented in the final section of the paper.

## COMPETENCIES AND LEARNING OBJECTIVES

The competencies and learning objectives related to the curricular content are as follows:

• To understand the framework for and major pieces of legislation and regulations in environmental and occupational health.
• To understand the potential and actual impacts of the workplace and general environment on the health of individual clients and communities in which nurses practice.
• To understand and be able to articulate the role of nursing practice in promoting environmental health.
• To demonstrate knowledge of the role of advocacy and justice in environmental health.
• To understand the principles behind how and why individuals perceive environmental risks as they do and to be able to incorporate these principles into a successful risk communication program.
• To understand the basic mechanism of exposure to environmental hazards.
• To demonstrate the ability to recognize and propose basic control strategies for common environmental hazards.
• To demonstrate the ability to recognize sentinel environmental illnesses.
• To demonstrate the ability to successfully complete an occupational and environmental health history.
• To demonstrate the ability to make a referral to a specialist practitioner or public health agency when a patient or group presents with a probable occupational or environmental etiology for their condition.

## SPECIALTY AREAS AND EDUCATIONAL LEVELS

The essential curricular content, competencies, and objectives described above are proposed for basic nursing curricula in general. It should be possible to integrate most, if not all, of the proposed content into existing course work. A more in-depth and comprehensive approach to this content is possible in a baccalaureate nursing program. An associate degree or diploma program has more constraints on its curriculum and very little focus on community health nursing. Specialty courses or electives offer additional opportunities for more in-depth learning in environmental health. Graduate education offers the opportunity for more advanced training in all of the content areas.

The following section contains recommendations for where to incorporate the proposed content into existing didactic course work. Note that in certain content areas the term *must* is used, whereas in other areas the term *should be* or *could be incorporated* is used. These terms were chosen to reflect the level of priority that the author believes is associated with incorporating the various elements of the content into existing curricula. Although no discussion of clinical or field experiences is included in this proposal, it should be highlighted that clinical experiences that incorporate these concepts and processes are essential for truly enhancing the environmental health content in nursing practice.

### Basic Nursing Education

— Legislation and regulations should be incorporated into existing leadership and/or policy course work. Principles of environmental advocacy could be taught in either leadership or community health course work. Environmental justice should be addressed in ethics and/or community health course work.

— Principles of toxicology (e.g., exposure and dose) should be incorporated into existing pharmacology course work. The effects of chemicals on organ systems (environmental illness) must be incorporated into pathophysiology and medical/surgery course work.

— Environmental and occupational history taking must be included in any physical assessment and/or nursing diagnosis course work.

— The impact of the environment and occupation on mental health and overall well-being should be incorporated into psycho-socio-cultural course work.

— Reproductive and childhood toxicants (e.g., prenatal and childhood lead exposure, pesticide exposure, and household chemical exposures) must be included within parent-child nursing course work.

— Hazard recognition and control should be included within existing community health course work.

### Specialty/Elective Course Work and Graduate Study

More advanced education in the above areas should be incorporated into the following elective course work and graduate education in these specialty areas:

— Objectives and time in public health, community health, and primary health care nursing course work must be dedicated to health concerns related to air, food, water, and soil quality.

— Parent–child and family course work must include lecture content on prenatal and childhood lead exposure, pesticide exposure, environmentally induced asthma, health effects of environmental tobacco smoke, and household chemical exposures.

— Women's health course work must include lecture content on chemical, physical, and biological agents suspected of being reproductive toxins. Emergency room or trauma course work must include injuries and illnesses resulting from toxic chemical exposures, in particular, emergency chemical releases.

— Medical/surgery course work must include lecture content on the health effects of chronic exposure to chemical, physical, and biological agents on the job and in the environment (e.g., asbestos, pesticides, heavy metals, solvents, and radon).

— Oncology course work must include content on environmentally caused (or suspected of causing) cancer.

— Neurology specialty course work must include content on neurological conditions related to acute and chronic solvent and other neurotoxin exposure.

Lastly, the author would recommend that all basic nursing education include content on the health hazards that nurses will face as health care professionals (e.g., chemotherapeutic agents, ethylene oxide, aerosolized drugs, tuberculosis, blood-borne pathogens, radiation, back injuries, stress, and shift work). Not only is this information critical to a successful career in nursing, but hazards in the health care setting can serve as very relevant case studies or examples for teaching the principles of hazard recognition and control.

# D
# Environmental Health Resources: Agencies, Organizations, Services, General References, and Tables of Environmental Health Hazards

**Contents**

# INTRODUCTION

For those interested in learning more about environmental health and the resources available that are related to environmental health, Appendix D presents names, addresses, and phone numbers of relevant government agencies and professional associations and organizations, as well as information about computerized information services, and a listing of general references. Agencies, associations, and organizations related to nursing and/or the environment are specifically highlighted. Finally, three tables are presented (pp. 214–240) that describe (1) selected environmental agents and their associated sources and potential exposures, (2) selected work-related diseases, disorders, and conditions associated with various agents, and (3) selected job categories, exposures, and associated work-related diseases and conditions for use in actual nursing practice.

The information presented in this appendix is not intended to be comprehensive or exhaustive, but rather supplemental and complementary.

# GOVERNMENT AGENCIES

Throughout our history, numerous federal and state agencies have been created to address the issues related to safety and health in the workplace, as well as the surrounding environment. Federal and state agencies have become increasingly involved in examining and monitoring the impact of the environment on the health of the public. The following list highlights several of the federal and state agencies currently involved in monitoring, evaluating, and protecting the environment and its relation to public health. Each agency is an invaluable source of information and can readily provide additional resources upon one's request. The agencies are listed in alphabetical order with federal organizations first, followed by state agencies.

## Federal Agencies

### *Agency for Toxic Substances and Disease Registry*

The Agency for Toxic Substances and Disease Registry (ATSDR) was created by Superfund legislation in 1980 as a part of the U.S. Department of Health and Human Services. ATSDR's mission is to prevent or mitigate adverse human health effects and diminished quality of life resulting from exposure to hazardous substances in the environment. In order to carry out its mission and to serve the needs of the American people, ATSDR conducts activities in public health assessments, health investigations, exposure and disease registry, emergency response, toxicological profiles, health education, and applied research.

ATSDR's Division of Health Education is mandated to assemble, develop, and distribute to the states, medical colleges, physicians, and other health professionals, educational materials on medical surveillance, screening, and methods of diagnosis and treatment of injury or disease related to exposure to hazardous substances. The Division also provides training and education for primary care physicians to diagnose and treat illness caused by hazardous substances and supports curriculum development and applied research in the area of environmental health.

The Division has developed a self-study series called Case Studies in Environmental Medicine which uses case studies to guide physicians through the diagnosis and treatment of illnesses related to hazardous substances exposure.

Several projects have also been developed and implemented to advance these goals. Some of the programs are described below:

- State Cooperative Agreements offer funding and assistance to state health departments for developing educational materials and activities in environmental medicine for health care professionals;
- National Association of County Health Officials Environmental Health Project is a cooperative agreement with ATSDR to conduct instructional sessions and develop supporting materials for local health officials and the medical community  concerning the communication of health risks from exposure to hazardous substances;
- Project EPOCH-Envi is co-sponsored by ATSDR and the National Institute for Occupational Safety and Health (NIOSH). Through the cooperative agreement, a consortium of medical schools works towards introducing curricula in occupational and environmental medicine in primary care residency programs;

Agency for Toxic Substances and Disease Registry
1600 Clifton Road, N.E.
Mail Stop E-28
Atlanta, GA 30333
(404) 639-0501
Emergencies (404) 639-0615

*Centers for Disease Control and Prevention*

The Centers for Disease Control and Prevention (CDC) is charged with protecting the public health of the nation by providing leadership and direction in the prevention and control of diseases and other prevent-able conditions and responding to public health emergencies.

Centers for Disease Control and Prevention
1600 Clifton Road, N.E.
Atlanta, GA 30333
(404) 639-3286

*Consumer Product Safety Commission*

The Consumer Products Safety Commission provides information on health and safety effects related to consumer products. It has direct juris-diction over chronic and chemical hazards in consumer products; assists consumers in evaluating the comparative safety of consumer products; develops uniform safety standards for consumer products and minimizes conflicting state and local regulations; and promotes research and investi-gation into the causes and prevention of product-related deaths, illnesses, and injuries.

Consumer Product Safety Commission
East West Towers
4340 East West Highway
Bethesda, MD 20814
(301) 504-0580
(800) 638-2772

*Department of Energy*

The Department of Energy (DOE) provides the framework for a com-prehensive and balanced national energy plan through the coordination and administration of the energy functions of the federal government. The Department is responsible for long-term, high-risk research and de-velopment of energy technology; the marketing of federal power; energy conservation; the nuclear weapons program; energy regulatory programs; and a central energy data collection and analysis program.

The Environment, Safety and Health Office of the DOE provides in-dependent oversight of departmental execution of environmental, occu-pational safety and health, and nuclear/nonnuclear safety and security laws, regulations, and policies; ensures that departmental programs are in compliance with environmental, health, and nuclear/nonnuclear safety protection plans, regulations, and procedures; provides an independent overview and assessment of Department-controlled activities to ensure that safety-impacted programs receive management review; and carries out legal functions of the nuclear safety civil penalty and criminal referral activities mandated by the Price-Anderson Amendments Act.

Department of Energy
1000 Independence Avenue, S.W.
Washington, DC 20585
(202) 586-5000

## Department of Health and Human Services

The Department of Health and Human Services (DHHS) is the Cabinet-level department of the federal executive branch most concerned with people and most involved with the nation's human concerns. In one way or another—whether it is mailing out social security checks or making health services more widely available—DHHS touches the lives of more Americans than any other federal agency. It is literally a department of people saving people, from newborn infants to our most elderly citizens.

Department of Health and Human Services
200 Independence Avenue, S.W.
Washington, DC 20201
(202) 679-0257

## Environmental Protection Agency

The Environmental Protection Agency (EPA) was established in 1970 in order to permit coordinated and effective governmental action on behalf of the environment. It endeavors to abate and control pollution systematically, by proper integration of a variety of research, monitoring, standard setting, and enforcement activities. As a complement to its other activities, the Agency coordinates and supports research and antipollution activities by state and local governments, private and public groups, individuals, and educational institutions. It also reinforces efforts among other federal agencies with respect to the impact of their operations on the environment, and it is specifically charged with publishing its determinations when those hold that a proposal is unsatisfactory from the standpoint of public health or welfare or environmental quality. In all, the EPA is designed to serve as the public's advocate for a livable environment.

Environmental Protection Agency
401 M Street, S.W.
Washington, DC 20460
(202) 260-2090

*Food and Drug Administration*

The Food and Drug Administration (FDA) inspects manufacturing plants and warehouses, collects and analyzes samples of foods, drugs, cosmetics, and therapeutic devices for adulteration and misbranding. Responsibilities also extend to sanitary preparation and handling of foods, waste disposal on interstate carriers, and enforcement of the Radiation Control Act as related to consumer products. Epidemiological and other investigations are conducted to determine causative factors or possible health hazards involved in adverse reactions or hazardous materials accidents. Investigators are located in resident posts in major cities throughout the country.

> Food and Drug Administration
> National Headquarters
> 200 C Street, S.W.
> Washington, DC  20204
> (301) 443-2410

*Health Resources and Services Administration*

Health Resources and Services Administration (HRSA) is responsible for general health services and resource issues relating to issues of access, equity, quality, and cost of care.  In order to accomplish this goal, the Administration supports states and communities in their efforts to deliver health care to underserved segments of the population; participates in the federal campaign against AIDS; provides leadership in improving the education, distribution, quality, and use of the health professionals needed to staff the nation's health care system; tracks the supply of and requirements for health professionals and addresses their competence through the development of a health practitioner data bank; and strengthens the public health system by working with state and local public health agencies.

> Health Resources and Services Administration
> 5600 Fishers Lane
> Rockville, MD 20857
> (301) 443-2086

*National Cancer Institute*

The National Cancer Institute (NCI) conducts and funds research on the causes, diagnosis, treatment, prevention, control, and biology of cancer and the rehabilitation of people with cancer. NCI also funds projects for innovative and effective approaches to preventing and controlling cancer, establishes multidisciplinary cancer care and clinical research activities in community hospitals, and supports cancer research training, clinical training, continuing education, and career development.

National Cancer Institute
National Institutes of Health
9000 Rockville Pike
Bethesda, MD 20892
(301) 496-5615
(800) 422-6237/(800) 4CANCER

*National Center for Environmental Health*

The mission of the National Center for Environmental Health (NCEH) is to promote health and quality of life by preventing or controlling disease, injury, and disability related to the interactions between people and their environment outside the workplace. To achieve these goals, NCEH directs programs both to prevent the adverse health effects of exposure to toxic substances and to combat the societal and environmental factors that increase the likelihood of exposure and disease. NCEH also works to prevent injuries and diseases resulting from natural or technologic disasters and to prevent birth defects and development disabilities resulting from nutritional deficiencies or exposure to environmental toxins in utero or during early childhood.

National Center for Environmental Health
Mailstop F29
4770 Buford Highway, N.E.
Atlanta, GA 30341-3724
(404) 488-7003

*National Institute for Occupational Safety and Health*

The National Institute for Occupational Safety and Health (NIOSH) was established by the Occupational Safety and Health Act of 1970 to conduct research on occupational diseases and injuries, respond to requests for assistance by investigating problems of health and safety in the workplace, recommend standards to the Occupational Safety and Health Administration (OSHA) and the Mine Safety and Health Administration (MSHA), and train professionals in occupational safety and health.

National Institute for Occupational Safety and Health
200 Independence Avenue, S.W.
Washington, DC 20201
(800) 356-4674

The NIOSH Technical Information Branch provides a toll-free technical information service (1-800-35-NIOSH) that provides convenient public access to NIOSH and its information resources. Callers may request information about NIOSH activities or about any aspect of occupational safety and health.

NIOSH Technical Information Branch
Robert A. Taft Laboratory
Mail Stop C-19
4676 Columbia Parkway
Cincinnati, OH 45226-1998
(800) 35-NIOSH

Project EPOCH-Envi. In conjunction with ATSDR, NIOSH established Project EPOCH-Envi to provide support and training to medical schools from around the country who wish to implement curricula in occupational and environmental medicine in primary care residency programs. Through this cooperative agreement, Project EPOCH-Envi conducts workshops and training programs for interested medical school faculty. The sessions focus on instructing faculty members how to develop curricula in occupational and environmental medicine.

Project EPOCH-Envi
National Institute for Occupational Safety and Health
Division of Training and Manpower Development
Curriculum Development Branch
Robert A. Taft Laboratories
4676 Columbia Parkway
Cincinnati, OH 45226-1998
(800) 356-4674

NIOSH Educational Resource Centers. The National Institute for Occupational Safety and Health (NIOSH) funds Educational Resource Centers (ERCs) which conduct research and administer graduate training programs in occupational medicine, occupational health nursing, and industrial hygiene and safety. They also provide continuing education programs for safety and health professionals and outreach programs for the community.

## ALABAMA
University of Alabama in
    Birmingham
School of Nursing
University of Starion
Birmingham, AL 35294-1210
Kathleen Brown, RN, Ph.D.
Director, Occupational Health
    Nursing
Degree: MSN, DNS
(205) 934-6858

## CALIFORNIA
UCLA School of Nursing
10833 LeConte Avenue
Los Angeles, CA 90024-1702
Linda Glazner, DrPH, RN
Program Director, Occupational
    Health Nursing
Degree: MSN
(310) 206-3838

University of California, San
    Francisco
School of Nursing
Department of Mental Health and
    Community Nursing N505Y
San Francisco, CA 94143
Julia Faucett, RN, Ph.D.
Program Director, Occupational
    Health Nursing
Degree: MS, DNS
(415) 476-5312

## ILLINOIS
University of Illinois at Chicago
College of Nursing
845 South Damen Street
Chicago, IL 60612
Karen Conrad, Ph.D., RN
Director, Occupational Health
    Nursing Program
Degree: MS, Ph.D.
(312) 996-7974

## MARYLAND
The Johns Hopkins University
School of Hygiene and Public
    Health
615 N. Wolfe Street
Baltimore, MD 21205
Jacqueline Agnew, RN, Ph.D.
Director, Occupational Health
    Nursing Program
Degree: MPH, DrPH, Ph.D.
(410) 955-4082

## MASSACHUSETTS
Harvard University
Harvard School of Public Health
Department of Environmental
    Science and Physiology
665 Huntington Avenue
Boston, MA 02115
Carol Love, Ph.D.
Director, Occupational Health
    Nursing (Simmons)
Degree: MS
(617) 738-2255

## MICHIGAN
University of Michigan
School of Nursing
Department of Community Health
    Nursing
400 N. Ingalls, Room 3340
Ann Arbor, MI 48109
Sally Lusk, RN, Ph.D.
Director, Occupational Health
    Nursing Program
Degree: MS
(313) 747-0347

**MINNESOTA**
University of Minnesota
School of Public Health
420 Delaware Street, SE, Box 197
Minneapolis, MN 55455
Patricia McGovern, RN, MPH
Program Director, Occupational
    Health Nursing
Degree: Ph.D., MS, MS/MPH
(612) 625-7429

**NEW YORK/NEW JERSEY**
University of Medicine and
    Dentistry of New Jersey
School of Nursing
30 Bergen Street
ADMC 119
Newark, NJ 07107-3000
Gail Buckler, RN, MPH, COHN
Program Director, OHN Program
Degree: MSN
(908) 445-0123

**NORTH CAROLINA**
University of North Carolina at
    Chapel Hill
School of Public Health
Rosenau Hall
Chapel Hill, NC 27514
Bonnie Rogers, RN, DrPH
Program Director, Occupational
    Health Nursing
Degree: MPH, MS
(919) 996-1030

**OHIO**
University of Cincinnati
College of Nursing and Health
200 Proctor Hall
3110 Vine
Cincinnati, OH 45219-0038
Sue Davis, Ph.D.
Acting Program Director,
    Occupational Health Nursing
Degree: MSN, Ph.D.
(513) 558-5280

**TEXAS**
University of Texas
The University of Texas Health
    Science Center at Houston
School of Public Health
P.O. Box 20186
Houston, TX 77225
Mary Kay Garcia, RN, DrPH
Director, Occupational Health for
    Nurses Program
Degree: MPH
(713) 792-7456

**UTAH**
University of Utah
RMCOEH, Building 512
Salt Lake City, UT 84119
Darlene Meservy, RN, MPH,
    DrPH
Director, Occupational Health
    Nursing
Degree: MSPH, Ph.D., MPH
(801) 581-8214

**WASHINGTON**
University of Washington
Community Health Care Systems,
   SM-24
Seattle, WA 98195
Mary Salazar, Ph.D.
Director, Occupational Health
   Nursing Program
Degree: MN, Ph.D., MN/MPH
(206) 685-0857

**Training Project Grants**
University of Pennsylvania
School of Nursing
420 Service Drive
Philadelphia, PA 19104
Winifred Hayes, RN, Ph.D.
Director, Occupational Health
   Nursing Program
Degree: MSN
(215) 898-1794

University of South Florida
College of Nursing
Health Science Center
Box 22
12901 Bruce B. Downs Boulevard
Tampa, FL 33612-4799
Dr. Candace Burns
Director, Occupational Health
   Nursing
Program
(813) 974-9160

*National Institute of Environmental Health Sciences*

   The National Institute of Environmental Health Sciences (NIEHS) is the principal federal agency for biomedical research on the effects of chemical, physical, and biological environmental agents on human health and well-being. The Institute supports research and training focused on the identification, assessment, and mechanism of action of potentially harmful agents in the environment. Research results form the basis for preventive programs for environmentally-related diseases and for action by regulatory agencies.

   The NIEHS currently sponsors several programs available to the medical school community, individual researchers, and other organizations or centers interested in studying the effects of the environment on health and how to better educate medical school students, employees, and the general public about environmental health risks and hazards. Some of the awards are described below:

   • The Environmental/Occupational Medicine Academic Award Program was established by the NIEHS to address the need for increased awareness by physicians of the impact of environmental and occupational conditions on illness, injury, and death. The award serves to assist in improving the quality of environmental/occupational medicine curricula and of fostering research careers in occupational medicine.

Environmental/Occupational Medicine Academic Awards
Chief, Environmental Health Resources Branch
Division of Extramural Research and Training
National Institute of Environmental Health Services
P.O. Box 12233
Research Triangle Park, NC 27709
(919) 541-7825

- Environmental Health Sciences Center Awards provide core support to universities for multidisplinary research in environmental health. Each center serves as national resources for environmental health research and manpower development. Areas of particular interest include: air, water, and food pollution; toxic mechanisms and body defense mechanisms; and the environmental aspects of cancer, birth defects, behavioral anomalies, respiratory and cardiovascular disease and diseases of other organs.
- Superfund Hazardous Substances–Basic Research and Education Program supports research to expand the base of scientific knowledge needed for adequate assessment of exposure and health risks from the release of hazardous substances, reduction in the amount and toxicity of hazardous substances, and ultimately, to prevent adverse human health effects.
- Hazardous Waste Worker Health and Safety Training provides grant support for the development and administration of health and safety training programs for workers and supervisors engaged in activities related to hazardous waste removal, containment, and transportation, or emergency response. In 1991, this program was expanded to include workers involved in generating and transporting hazardous materials and wastes, oil spill cleanup workers, and workers involved in the cleanup of nuclear workshops facilities.
- Clinical Investigator Award provides for the development of clinical investigators in the field of environmental health/human toxicology. The award of up to $35,000 per year supports the research development of physicians to work with research teams on problems arising from the exposures of human populations to environmental chemicals.

National Institute of Environmental Health Sciences
P.O. Box 12233
104 T.W. Alexander Drive
Research Triangle Park, NC 27709
(919) 541-3212

## National Institutes of Health

The National Institutes of Health (NIH) is the principal biomedical research agency of the federal government. Its mission is to pursue knowledge to improve human health. To accomplish this goal, the Institute seeks to expand fundamental knowledge about the nature and behavior of living systems, to apply that knowledge to extend the health of human lives, and to reduce the burdens resulting from disease and disability. In the quest of this mission, NIH supports biomedical and behavioral research around the world, trains promising young researchers, and promotes the acquisition and distribution of medical knowledge. Research activities conducted by NIH will determine much of the quality of health care for the future and reinforce the quality of health care currently available.

National Institutes of Health
9000 Rockville Pike
Bethesda, MD 20892

## National Institute of Nursing Research

The National Institute of Nursing Research (NINR) provides leadership for nursing research, supports and conducts research and training, and disseminates information to build a scientific base for nursing practice and patient care, and to promote health and improve the effects of illness on the general public. NINR also provides grants and awards for nursing research and research training. Programs include research in health promotion and disease prevention, acute and chronic illness, and delivery of nursing care.

National Institute of Nursing Research
9000 Rockville Pike
Building 31 #5803
Bethesda, MD 20892
(301) 496-0207

*Nuclear Regulatory Commission*

The Nuclear Regulatory Commission (NRC) licenses and regulates civilian use of nuclear energy to protect health and safety and the environment. This is achieved by licensing persons and companies to build and operate nuclear reactors and other facilities and to own and use nuclear materials. The Commission makes rules and sets standards for these types of licenses. It also carefully inspects the activities of the persons and companies licensed to ensure that they do not violate the safety rules of the Commission.

Nuclear Regulatory Commission
Washington, DC 20555
(301) 492-7000

*Occupational Safety and Health Administration*

The Occupational Safety and Health Administration (OSHA) was created within the Department of Labor under the Occupational Safety and Health Act of 1970 to enforce national occupational health and safety standards. OSHA encourages employers and employees to reduce workplace hazards, implements new or improved safety and health programs, provides research in occupational safety and health, requires a reporting and recording system to monitor job-related illnesses and injuries, training, develops mandatory job safety and health standards and enforces them effectively, and provides for the development, analysis, evaluation, and approval of state occupational safety and health programs.

Occupational Safety and Health Administration
Office of Administrative Services
200 Constitution Avenue, N.W.
Room N-310
Washington, DC 20210
(202) 219-4667

## State Agencies

*State Health Departments and Radon Contacts*

**Alabama Department of Public Health**
434 Monroe Street
Montgomery, AL 36130
(205) 242-5052
Radon: Montgomery
(800) 582-1866
(205) 242-5315

**Alaska Division of Public Health**
Department of Health and Social
    Services
P.O. Box H
Juneau, AK 99811
(907) 465-3090
Radon: Juneau
(800) 478-4845
(907) 465-3019

**Arizona Department of Health Services**
1740 W. Adams Street
Phoenix, AZ 85007
(602) 542-1024
Radon: Phoenix
(602) 255-4845

**Arkansas Department of Health**
4815 W. Markham Street
Little Rock, AR 72205
(501) 661-2111
Radon: Little Rock
(501) 661-2301

**California Department of Health Services**
714 P Street
Sacramento, CA 95814
(916) 657-1425
Radon: Sacramento
(916) 324-2208

**Colorado Department of Health**
4210 E. 11th Avenue
Denver, CO 80220
(303) 331-4600
Radon: Denver
(800) 846-3986
(303) 692-3057

**Connecticut Department of Health Services**
150 Washington Street
Hartford, CT 06106
(203) 566-2038
Radon: Hartford
(203) 566-3122

**Delaware Division of Public Health**
Department of Health and Social
    Services
P.O. Box 637
Dover, DE 19903
(302) 739-4701
Radon: Dover
(302) 739-3787
(800) 554-4636 (In-state)

**District of Columbia Department of Human Services**
Commission of Public Health
1660 L Street, N.W., 12th Floor
Washington, DC 20036
(202) 673-7700
Radon: Washington, DC
(202) 727-7221

**Florida Health Office**
Department of Health and
 Rehabilitation Services
1323 Winewood Blvd.
Building 1
Tallahassee, FL 32301
(904) 487-2705
Radon: Orlando
(904) 488-1525
(800) 543-8279

**Georgia Division of Public Health**
878 Peachtree Street
Atlanta, GA 30309
(404) 894-7505
Radon: Atlanta
(404) 894-6644

**Guam Public Health and Social Services**
P.O. Box 2816
Agana, Guam 96910
(671) 734-2083
Hawaii Department of Health
1250 Punchbowl Street
P.O. Box 3378
Honolulu, HI 96801
(808) 586-4410
Radon: Honolulu
(808) 543-4383

**Idaho Division of Health**
Department of Health and Welfare
450 W. State Street
Boise, ID 83720
(208) 334-5945
Radon: Boise
(800) 445-8647
(208) 334-6584

**Illinois Department of Public Health**
535 W. Jefferson Street
Springfield, IL 62761
(217) 782-4977
Radon: Springfield
(800) 325-1245
(217) 786-6384

**Indiana Board of Health**
P.O. Box 1964
1330 W. Michigan Street
Indianapolis, IN 46206
(317) 633-8400
Radon: Indianapolis
(317) 633-0150
(800) 272-9723 (In-state)

**Iowa Department of Public Health**
Robert Lucas State
 Office Building
East 12th and Walnut Streets
Des Moines, IA 50319
(515) 281-5605
Radon: Des Moines
(515) 281-7781
(800) 383-5992 (In-state)

**Kansas Department of Health and Environment**
900 SW Jackson
Topeka, KS 66612
(913) 296-1522
Radon: Topeka
(913) 296-1560

**Kentucky Department for Health Services**
Cabinet for Human Resources
275 E. Main Street
Frankfort, KY 40621
(502) 564-3970
Radon: Frankfort
(502) 564-3700

**Louisiana Department of Health and Hospitals**
P.O. Box 629
Baton Rouge, LA 70821
(504) 342-9500
Radon: Baton Rouge
(800) 256-2494
(504) 925-7042

**Maine Bureau of Health**
Department of Human Services
State House Station 11
Augusta, ME 04333
(207) 289-2736
Radon: Augusta
(800) 232-0842
(207) 789-5689

**Maryland Department of Health and Mental Hygiene**
201 W. Preston Street
Baltimore, MD 21201
(301) 225-6500
Radon: Baltimore
(800) 872-3666
(301) 631-3300

**Massachusetts Department of Public Health**
150 Tremont Street
Boston, MA 02111
(617) 727-2700
Radon: North Hampton
(413) 586-7525

**Michigan Department of Public Health**
3423 N. Logan Street
Lansing, MI 48909
(517) 335-8024.
Radon: Lansing
(517) 335-8190

**Minnesota Department of Health**
717 Delaware Street, S.E.
P.O. Box 9441
Minneapolis, MN 55440
(612) 623-5460
Radon: Minneapolis
(612) 627-5012
(800) 798-9050

**Mississippi Department of Health**
P.O. Box 1700
2423 N. State Street
Jackson, MS 39215
(601) 960-7634
Radon: Jackson
(800) 626-7739
(601) 354-6657

**Missouri Department of Health**
P.O. Box 570
Jefferson City, MO 65102
(314) 751-60001
Radon: Jefferson City
(314) 751-6083
(800) 669-7236 (In-state)

**Montana Department of Health and Environmental Sciences**
Cogswell Building
Helena, MT 59620
(406) 444-2544
Radon: Helena
(406) 444-3671

**Nebraska Department of Health**
301 Centennial Mall S.
P.O. Box 95007
Lincoln, NE 68509
(402) 471-4047
Radon: Lincoln
(402) 471-2168
(800) 334-9491 (In-state)

**Nevada Health Division**
505 E. King Street
Carson City, NV 89710
(702) 687-4740
Radon: Carson City
(702) 687-5394

**New Hampshire Division of Public Health Services**
Health and Welfare Building
Hazen Drive
Concord, NH 03301
(603) 271-4500
Radon: Concord
(603) 271-4674

**New Jersey Department of Health**
CN 360
Trenton, NJ 08625
(609) 292-7837
Radon: Trenton
(609) 987-6396
(800) 648-0394

**New Mexico Health and Environmental Department**
1190 South Francis Drive
Santa Fe, NM 87503
(505) 827-2613
Radon: Santa Fe
(505) 827-4300

**New York Department of Health**
Tower Building
Empire State Plaza
Albany, NY 12237
(518) 474-2011
Radon: Albany
(518) 458-6451

**North Carolina Department of Environment**
Health and Natural Resources
Division of Health Services
P.O. Box 27687
Raleigh, NC 27611
(919) 733-4984
Radon: Raleigh
(919) 571-4141

**North Dakota Department of Health and Consolidated Labs**
State Capitol Judicial Wing
600 E. Boulevard Avenue
Bismarck, ND 58505
(701) 224-2372
Radon: Bismarck
(701) 224-2348

**Ohio Department of Health**
246 N. High Street
Columbus, OH 43266
(614) 466-2253
Radon: Columbus
(614) 644-2727
(800) 523-4439 (In-state)

**Oklahoma Department of Health**
1000 NE 10th Street
P.O. Box 53551
Oklahoma City, OK 73152
(405) 271-4200
Radon: Oklahoma City
(405) 271-5221

**Oregon State Health Division**
1400 SW 5th Avenue
Portland, OR 97201
(503) 229-4032
Radon: Portland
(503) 731-4014

**Pennsylvania Department of Health**
P.O. Box 90
Harrisburg, PA 17108
(717) 787-6436
Radon: Harrisburg
(717) 787-2480
(800) 23-RADON (In-state)

**Puerto Rico Department of Health**
Building A, Call Box 70184
San Juan, PR 00936
(809) 766-1616
Radon: Rio Piedras
(809) 767-3563

**Rhode Island Department of Health**
Cannon Health Building
3 Capitol Hill
Providence, RI 02908
(401) 277-2231
Radon: Providence
(401) 277-2438

**South Carolina Department of Health and Environmental Control**
2600 Bull Street
Columbia, SC 29201
(803) 735-4880
Radon: Columbia
(800) 768-0362
(803) 734-4700

**South Dakota Department of Health**
445 E. Capitol
Pierre, SD 57501
(605) 773-3361
Radon: Pierre
(605) 773-3351

**Tennessee Department of Health and Environment**
344 Cordell Hull Building
Nashville, TN 37247-0101
(615) 741-3111
Radon: Nashville
(800) 232-1139
(615) 741-3651

**Texas Department of Health**
1100 W. 49th Street
Austin, TX 78756
(512) 458-7111
Radon: Austin
(512) 834-6688

**Utah Department of Health**
288 N. 1460 W.
P.O. Box 16700
Salt Lake City, UT 84116
(801) 538-6111
Radon: Salt Lake City
(801) 538-6734

**Vermont Department of Health**
P.O. Box 70
60 Main Street
Burlington, VT 05402
(802) 863-7280
Radon: Montpelier
(800) 640-0601
(802) 828-2886

**Virgin Island Department of Health**
L18 Sugar Estate
St. Thomas, VI 00802
(809) 774-4888

**Virginia Department of Health**
P.O. Box 2448
Richmond, VA 23218
(804) 786-3561
Radon: Richmond
(800) 468-0138
(804) 786-5932

**Washington Department of Health**
1112 S.E. Quince Street
Olympia, WA 98504-7890
(206) 753-5871
Radon: Olympia
(800) 323-9727
(206) 753-4518

**West Virginia Department of Public Health**
Building 3, State Capital Complex
Charleston, WV 25305
(304) 348-2971
Radon: South Charleston
(304) 558-3526
(800) 922-1255 (In-state)

**Wisconsin Division of Health**
Department of Health and Social
  Services
P.O. Box 309
Madison, WI 53707
(608) 266-1511
Radon: Madison
(608) 267-4795

**Wyoming Health and Medical Services**
Hathaway Building
Cheyenne, WY 82002
(307) 777-6464
Radon: Cheyenne
(800) 458-5847
(307) 777-6015

*Environmental Council of States (ECOS Member States Directory)*

**ALABAMA**
John Smith
Director
Alabama Department of
  Environmental Management
1751 Congressman W.L. Dickinson
  Drive
P.O. Box 371463
Montgomery, AL 36130-1463
(334) 271-7761

**ALASKA**
Gene Burden
Commissioner
Alaska Department of
  Environmental
Conservation
410 Willoughby Avenue, Suite 105
Juneau, AK 99801-1795
(907) 465-5066

**ARIZONA**
Edward Z. Fox
Director
Arizona Department of
    Environmental Quality
3033 N. Central Avenue
Phoenix, AZ 85012
(602) 207-2203

**ARKANSAS**
Randall Mathis
Director
Arkansas Department of Pollution
    Control and Ecology
8001 National Drive
P.O. Box 8913
Little Rock, AR 72219-8913
(501) 570-2130

**CALIFORNIA**
James M. Strock
Secretary
California Environmental
    Protection Agency
555 Capitol Mall, Suite 235
Sacramento, CA 95814
(916) 445-3846

**COLORADO**
Tom Looby
Director, Office of Environment
Colorado Department of Public
    Health and Environment
4300 Cherry Creek Drive, South
Denver, CO 80222
(303) 692-3001

**CONNECTICUT**
Sidney Holbrook
Commissioner
Connecticut Department of
    Environmental Protection
165 Capitol Avenue, Room 161
Hartford, CT 06106
(203) 424-3001

**DELAWARE**
Christophe A.G. Tulou
Secretary
Delaware Department of Natural
    Resources and Environmental
    Control
P.O. Box 1401
Dover, DE 19903
(302) 739-4403

**DISTRICT OF COLUMBIA**
Ferial Bishop
Administrator
District of Columbia
    Environmental Regulation
    Administration
2100 Martin Luther King, Jr.
    Avenue
Suite 203
Washington, DC 20020
(202) 645-6617

**FLORIDA**
Virginia B. Wetherell
Secretary
Florida Department of
    Environmental Protection
3900 Commonwealth Boulevard
Tallahassee, FL 32399
(904) 488-4805

## GEORGIA
Harold F. Reheis
Director, Environmental
    Protection Division
Georgia Department of Natural
    Resources
205 Butler Street, SE, Suite 1152
Atlanta, GA  30334
(404) 656-4713

## HAWAII
Bruce Anderson
Director for Environmental Health
P.O. Box 3378
Honolulu, HI  96801
(808) 586-4424

## IDAHO
Wallace Cory
Administrator
Idaho Division of Environmental
    Quality
450 W. State Street
Boise, ID  83720
(208) 334-5840

## ILLINOIS
Mary Gade
Director
Illinois Environmental Protection
    Agency
2200 Churchill Road
Springfield, IL  62706
(217) 782-9540

## INDIANA
Kathy Prosser
Commissioner
Indiana Department of
    Environmental
    Management
100 North Senate Avenue
P.O. Box 6015
Indianapolis, IN  46206-6015
(317) 232-8162

## KANSAS
Ron Hammerschmidt
Director, Division of Environment
Kansas Department of Health and
    Environment
740 Forbes Field
Topeka, KS  66620
(913) 296-1535

## KENTUCKY
Phillip J. Shepherd
Secretary
Kentucky Natural Resources and
    Environment
    Protection Cabinet
Capital Plaza Tower, 5th Floor
Frankfort, KY  40601
(502) 564-3350

## LOUISIANA
William Kucharski
Secretary
Louisiana Department of
    Environmental Quality
P.O. Box 82263
Baton Rouge, LA  70884-2263
(504) 765-0639

**MAINE**
Edward Sullivan
Commissioner
Maine Department of
    Environmental Protection
State House Station 17
Augusta, ME  04333
(207) 287-2812

**MARYLAND**
Jane T. Nishida
Secretary
Maryland Department of the
    Environment
2500 Broening Highway
Baltimore, MD  21224
(410) 631-3084

John Chlada
Director
Strategic Planning and
    Enforcement
Maryland Department of the
    Environment
2500 Broening Highway
Baltimore, MD  21224
(410) 631-3114

**MASSACHUSETTS**
David B. Strubs
Commissioner
Massachusetts Department of
    Environmental Protection
1 Winter Street
Boston, MA  02108
(617) 292-5856

**MICHIGAN**
Russell Harding
Deputy Director
Michigan Department of Natural
    Resources
P.O. Box 30028
Lansing, MI  48909
(517) 373-7917

**MINNESOTA**
Charles Williams
Commissioner
Minnesota Pollution Control
    Agency
520 Lafayette Road North
St. Paul, MN  55155-4194
(612) 296-7301

**MISSISSIPPI**
J.I. Palmer
Executive Director
Mississippi Department of
    Environmental
    Quality
P.O. Box 20305
2380 Highway 80 West
Jackson, MS  39289-1305
(601) 961-5000

**MISSOURI**
David A. Shorr
Director
Missouri Department of Natural
    Resources
P.O. Box 176
Jefferson City, MO  65102
(314) 751-4732

**NEBRASKA**
Randolph Wood
Director
Nebraska Department of
   Environmental
   Quality
P.O. Box 98922
Lincoln, NE 68509
(402) 471-4231

**NEW HAMPSHIRE**
Robert W. Varney
Commissioner
New Hampshire Department of
   Environmental Services
6 Hazen Drive
P.O. Box 95
Concord, NH 03301
(603) 271-3503

**NEW JERSEY**
Robert Shinn
New Jersey Department of
   Environmental
   Protection
401 E. State Street, CN 402
Trenton, NJ 08625
(609) 292-2885

**NEW MEXICO**
Mark Weidler
Secretary
New Mexico Environment
   Department
P.O. Box 26110
Santa Fe, NM 87502
(505) 827-2855

**NEW YORK**
Michael Zagata
Commissioner
New York Department of
   Environmental Conservation
50 Wolf Road
Albany, NY 12233-1010
(518) 457-1162

**NORTH CAROLINA**
Jonathon Howes
Secretary
North Carolina Department of
   Environment, Health and
   Natural Resources
P.O. Box 27687
Raleigh, NC 27611-7687
(919) 733-4984

**NORTH DAKOTA**
Francis Schwindt
Chief
North Dakota Environmental
   Health Section
1200 Missouri Avenue
P.O. Box 5520
Bismarck, ND 58502-5520
(701) 328-5150

**OHIO**
Donald R. Schregardus
Director
Ohio Environmental Protection
   Agency
1800 Watermark Drive
Columbus, OH 43266
(614) 644-2782

**OKLAHOMA**
Mark Coleman
Executive Director
Oklahoma Department of
    Environmental
    Quality
1000 NE 10th Street, Suite 1212
Oklahoma City, OK  73119-1212
(405) 271-8056

**OREGON**
Langdon Marsh
Director
Oregon Department of
    Environmental Quality
811 SW 6th Avenue
Portland, OR  97204
(503) 229-5696

**PENNSYLVANIA**
James Seif
Secretary
Pennsylvania Department of
    Environmental Resources
P.O. Box 2063
Harrisburg, PA  17105-2063
(717) 772-2724

**PUERTO RICO**
Hector Russe Martinez
Chairman
Puerto Rico Environmental
    Quality Board
P.O. Box 11488
San Juan, PR 00910
(809) 767-8056

**RHODE ISLAND**
Timothy R.E. Keeney
Director
Rhode Island Department of
    Environmental Management
9 Hayes Street
Providence, RI  02908
(401) 277-2234

**SOUTH CAROLINA**
R. Lewis Shaw
Deputy Commissioner
South Carolina Environmental
    Quality Control Division
2600 Bull Street
Columbia, SC  29201
(803) 734-5360

**SOUTH DAKOTA**
Nettie H. Meyers
Secretary
South Dakota Department of
    Environment and Natural
    Resources
Joe Foss Building
523 E. Capitol Avenue
Pierre, SD  57501
(605) 773-5559

**TENNESSEE**
J.W. Luna
Commissioner
Tennessee Department of
    Environment and
    Conservation
21st Floor, L & C Tower
401 Church Street
Nashville, TN  37243-0435
(615) 532-0109

**TEXAS**
Peggy Garner
Commissioner
Texas National Resource and
    Conservation Commission
P.O. Box 13087
Austin, TX 78711-3087
(512) 239-5515

**UTAH**
Brent C. Bradford
Deputy Director
Utah Department of
    Environmental Quality
P.O. Box 144810
Salt Lake City, UT 84114-4810
(801) 536-4405

**VERMONT**
Bill Brierley
Acting Commissioner
Vermont Agency of Natural
    Resources
103 S. Main Street, Building 1,
    South
Waterbury, VT 05671
(802) 241-3800

**WASHINGTON**
Mary Riveland
Director
Washington Department of
    Ecology
P.O. Box 47600
Olympia, WA 98504-7600
(206) 407-7001

**WISCONSIN**
George E. Meyer
Secretary
Wisconsin Department of Natural
    Resources
P.O. Box 7921
Madison, WI 53707
(608) 266-2121

**WYOMING**
Dennis Hemmer
Director
Wyoming Department of
    Environmental Quality
122 W. 25th Street
Cheyenne, WY 82002
(307) 777-7938

## ASSOCIATIONS AND ORGANIZATIONS

### American Academy of Nurse Practitioners

The American Academy of Nurse Practitioners (AANP) was established to promote high standards of health care delivered by nurse practitioners. AANP acts as a forum to enhance the identity and continuity of nurse practitioners while also addressing national and state legislative issues that affect its members.

American Academy of Nurse Practitioners
OBJ Building
P.O. Box 12846, Capital Station
Austin, TX 78711
(512) 442-4262

## American Academy of Nursing

The American Academy of Nursing (ANA) was established in order to help facilitate the advance of new concepts in nursing and health care. ANA attempts to identify and explore issues in health, the professions, and society that concern nursing, while also examining the interrelationships among the segments within nursing and the interaction among nurses as they affect the development of the nursing profession.

American Academy of Nursing
600 Maryland Avenue, S.W.
Suite 100 W
Washington, DC 20024-2571
(202) 554-4444

## American Assembly for Men in Nursing

The American Assembly for Men in Nursing (AAMN) was originally established to help eliminate prejudice in nursing for men. Today, the AAMN provides a forum for discussion of common problems, provides incentives for continuing education and professional growth, while also furthering the need for all health professionals to be sensitive to various social needs in the pursuit of positive health care.

American Assembly for Men in Nursing
P.O. Box 31753
Independence, OH 44131
(216) 524-3504

## American Association of Colleges of Nursing

The American Association of Colleges of Nursing (AACN) encompasses all institutions offering baccalaureate and/or graduate degrees in nursing. AACN seeks to advance the practice of professional nursing by improving the quality of educational programs offered, promoting research and developing academic leaders. AACN also works with other professional nursing organizations and organizations in the health professions to evaluate and improve health care.

American Association of Colleges of Nursing
1 Dupont Circle, N.W.
Washington, DC 20036
(202) 463-6930

## American Association of Occupational Health Nurses

The American Association of Occupational Health Nurses (AAOHN) is an organization of registered professional nurses employed by business and industrial firms; nurse educators, nurse editors, nurse writers; and others interested in occupational health nursing.

American Association of Occupational Health Nurses
50 Lenox Pointe
Atlanta, GA 30324
(800) 241-8014
(404) 262-1162

## American Association of Poison Control Centers

The American Association of Poison Control Centers (AAPCC) aids in the procurement of information on the ingredients and potential acute toxicity of substances that may cause accidental poisonings and on the proper management of such poisonings. The AAPCC has established standards for the poison information and control centers, offering immediate information through hotlines around the country. The AAPCC also conducts educational programs and prepares visual aids on prevention of accidental poisonings; maintains a national poisoning database; and operates a nationwide speakers' bureau.

American Association of Poison Control Centers
3800 Reservoir Road, N.W.
Washington, DC 20007
(202) 784-4666/362-7217
(202) 784-2530 FAX

**ALABAMA**
Birmingham
  Regional Poison Control
    Center
  The Children's Hospital of
    Alabama
  Emergency (205) 939-9201
  (800) 292-6678 (In-state)
  (205) 933-4050

**ARIZONA**
Phoenix
  Samaritan Regional Poison
    Center
  (602) 253-3334

Tucson
  Arizona Poison and Drug
    Information Center
  Emergency (800) 362-0101 (In-
    state)
  (602) 626-6016

## CALIFORNIA
Fresno
    Fresno Regional Poison
        Control Center
    Valley Children's Hospital
    Emergency (800) 346-5922 (In-
        state)
    (202) 445-1222

Sacramento
    University of California,
        Davis
    Medical Center Regional
        Poison Control Center
    Emergency (916) 734-3692
    (800) 342-9293 (In-state)

San Diego
    San Diego Regional Poison
        Control Center
    University of California, San
        Diego Medical Center
    Emergency (619) 543-6000
    (800) 876-4766 (In-state)

San Francisco
    San Francisco Bay Area
        Regional Poison Control
        Center
    San Francisco General
        Hospital
    Emergency (800) 523-2222

San Jose
    Santa Clara Valley Medical
        Center Regional Poison
        Center
    Emergency (408) 299-5112
    (800) 342-9293 (In-state)

## COLORADO
Denver
    Rocky Mountain Poison and
        Drug Center
    Emergency (303) 629-1123

## DISTRICT OF COLUMBIA
Washington
    National Capital Poison
        Control Center
    Georgetown University
        Hospital
    Emergency (202) 625-3333
    (202) 784-4660 (TTY)

## FLORIDA
Tampa
    The Florida Poison
        Information Center and
        Toxicology Resource
        Center
    Tampa General Hospital
    Emergency (813) 253-444
    (800) 282-3171 (In-state)

## GEORGIA
Atlanta
    Georgia Poison Center
    Grady Memorial Hospital
    Emergency (800) 282-5846 (In-
        state)
    (404) 616-9000

## INDIANA
Indianapolis
    Indiana Poison Center
    Methodist Hospital of Indiana
    Emergency (800) 382-9097 (In-
        state)
    (317) 929-2323

## MARYLAND
Baltimore
    Maryland Poison Center
    Emergency (410) 528-7701
    (800) 492-2414 (In-state)

## MASSACHUSETTS
Boston
    Massachusetts Poison Control
        System
    Emergency (617) 232-2120
    (800) 682-9211

## MICHIGAN
Detroit
    Poison Control Center
    Emergency (313) 745-5711

## MINNESOTA
Minneapolis
    Hennepin Regional Poison
        Center
    Hennepin County Medical
        Center
    Emergency (612) 347-3141
    (612) 337-7474 (TTY)

## MISSOURI
St. Louis
    Cardinal Glennon Children's
        Hospital
    Regional Poison Center
    Emergency (314) 772-5200
    (800) 366-8888 (In-state)

## MONTANA
Denver (Colorado)
    Rocky Mountain Poison and
        Drug Center
    Emergency (303) 629-1123

## NEBRASKA
Omaha
    The Poison Center
    Emergency (402) 390-5555
    (800) 955-9119 (In-state)

## NEW JERSEY
Newark
    New Jersey Poison
        Information and Education
        System
    Emergency (800) 962-1253 (In-state)

## NEW MEXICO
Albuquerque
    New Mexico Poison and Drug
        Information Center
    Emergency (505) 843-2551
    (800) 432-6866 (In-state)

## NEW YORK
Mineola
    Long Island Regional Poison
        Control Center
    Winthrop University Hospital
    Emergency (516) 542-2323

New York
    New York City Poison Control
        Center
    New York City Department of
        Health
    Emergency (212) 340-4494
    (212) P-O-I-S-O-N-S
    (212) 689-9014 (TDD)

Nyack
    Hudson Valley Poison Center
    Nyack Hospital
    Emergency (800) 336-6997
    (914) 353-1000

**OHIO**
Columbus
　　Central Ohio Poison Center
　　Emergency (614) 228-1323
　　(800) 682-7625
　　(614) 228-2272 (TTY)

Cincinnati
　　Cincinnati Drug and Poison
　　　Information Center and
　　　Regional Poison Control
　　　System
　　Emergency (513) 558-5111
　　(800) 872-5111

**OREGON**
Portland
　　Oregon Poison Center
　　Oregon Health Sciences
　　　University
　　Emergency (503) 494-8968
　　(800) 452-7165 (In-state)

**PENNSYLVANIA**
Philadelphia
　　The Poison Control Center
　　One Children's Center
　　Emergency (215) 386-2100

Pittsburgh
　　Pittsburgh Poison Center
　　Emergency (412) 681-6669

Hershey
　　Central Pennsylvania Poison
　　　Center
　　Milton S. Hershey Medical
　　　Center
　　Emergency (800) 521-6110

**RHODE ISLAND**
Providence
　　Rhode Island Poison Center
　　Emergency (401) 277-5727
　　(401) 277-8062 (TDD)

**TEXAS**
Dallas
　　North Texas Poison Center
　　Emergency (214) 590-5000
　　(800) 441-0040 (In-state)

Galveston
　　Texas State Poison Center
　　The University of Texas
　　　Medical Branch
　　Emergency (409) 765-1420
　　(713) 654-1701 (Houston)
　　(512) 478-4490 (Austin)

**UTAH**
Salt Lake City
　　Utah Poison Control Center
　　Emergency (801) 581-2151
　　(800) 456-7707 (In-state)

**VIRGINIA**
Charlottesville
　　Blue Ridge Poison Center
　　Emergency (804) 924-5543
　　(800) 451-1428

Northern Virginia
　　National Capital Poison
　　　Center
　　Georgetown University
　　　Hospital
　　Emergency (202) 625-3333
　　(202) 784-4660 (TTY)

**WEST VIRGINIA**
Charleston
West Virginia Poison Center
 Emergency (800) 642-3625 (In-
  state)
 (304) 348-4211

**WYOMING**
Omaha (Nebraska)
 The Poison Center
 Emergency (402) 390-5555
 (800) 955-9199 (NE and WY
  only)

### American Board for Occupational Health Nurses

The American Board for Occupational Health Nurses (ABOHN) establishes standards and confers initial and ongoing certification in occupational health nurses. Besides conducting annual certification examinations, the ABOHN awards occupational health nurses for excellence in the field and in research. The ABOHN has also created a database with information and directories relevant to occupational health and nursing.

American Board for Occupational Health Nurses
10503 N. Cedarburg Road
Mequon, WI 53092-4403
(414) 242-0704

### American Cancer Society

The American Cancer Society (ACS) is comprised of volunteers who support education and research in cancer prevention, diagnosis, detection, and treatment. ACS provides special services to cancer patients while also establishing educational programs for health professionals and communities.

American Cancer Society
1599 Clifton Road, N.E.
Atlanta, GA 30329
(800) ACS-2345

### American College of Obstetricians and Gynecologists

The American College of Obstetricians and Gynecologists (ACOG) is dedicated to the advancement of women's health through education, advocacy, practice, and research. ACOG works to serve as a strong advocate for quality health care for women, maintain the highest standards of clinical practice and continuing education for its members, promote patient education and stimulate patient understanding of, and involvement in, medical care, and increase awareness among its members and the public of the changing issues facing women's health care.

American College of Obstetricians and Gynecologists
409 12th Street, S.W.
Washington, DC 20024
(202) 638-5577

## American College of Occupational and Environmental Medicine

The American College of Occupational and Environmental Medicine (ACOEM) is an association of approximately 6,500 physicians attempting to educate members and other physicians, employers, other organizations, and the public-at-large about occupational and environmental health. The ACOEM has developed a continuing education course entitled *Core Curriculum in Environmental Medicine* in order to enhance physicians' critical thinking on environmental issues, improve their problem-solving skills, and make them more effective at decision-making about environmental concerns. Once the *Curriculum* has been fully developed, ACOEM will make the teaching materials available to other organizations, including medical schools. The ultimate goal of this project has been to enable health professionals to serve as environmental educators to all of the communities in which they are involved.

American College of Occupational and Environmental Medicine
55 West Seegers Road
Arlington Heights, IL 60005
(708) 228-6850

## American Lung Association

The American Lung Association (ALA) is a federation of state and local associations of physicians, nurses, and laymen interested in the prevention and control of lung disease. The Association works with other organizations in planning and conducting programs in community services, public, professional, and patient education, and research. The ALA also makes recommendations regarding medical care of respiratory disease, occupational health, hazards of smoking, and air conservation.

American Lung Association
1740 Broadway
New York, NY 10019-4374
(212) 315-8700

## American Nurses Association

The American Nurses Association (ANA) is comprised of registered nurses from around the country. ANA seeks to promote the nursing profession through its sponsorship of the American Nurses Foundation (for research), American Academy of Nursing, Center for Ethics and Human Rights, International Nursing Center, Ethnic/Racial Minority Fellowship Programs, and the American Nurses Credentialing Center.

American Nurses Association
600 Maryland Avenue, S.W.
Suite 100 W
Washington, DC 20024-2571
(202) 554-4444

## American Nurses Foundation

The American Nurses Foundation (ANF) was established by the American Nurses Association to conduct health policy research as it relates to nursing and the health care of the general public.

American Nurses Foundation
600 Maryland Avenue, S.W.
Suite 100 W
Washington, DC 20024-2571
(202) 554-4444

## American Public Health Association

The American Public Health Association (APHA) was founded in 1872 as a professional organization of physicians, nurses, educators, academicians, environmentalists, epidemiologists, new professionals, social workers, health administrators, optometrists, podiatrists, pharmacists, dentists, nutritionists, health planners, other community and mental health specialists, and any interested consumer. The APHA seeks to protect and promote personal, mental, and environmental health through the promulgation of health standards, establishment of uniform practices and procedures, development of etiology of communicable diseases, research in public health, exploration of medical care programs and their relationships to public health.

American Public Health Association
1015 15th Street, N.W.
Washington, DC 20005
(202) 789-5600

## Association of Black Nursing Faculty

The Association of Black Nursing Faculty (ABNF) is made up of black nursing faculty teaching in nursing programs accredited by the National League for Nursing. ABNF works to promote health-related issues and educational concerns of interest to the black community by providing forums for communication and the exchange of information among members, develops strategies to address the concerns of the community, and promotes health-related issues of legislation, government programs, and community activities.

Association of Black Nursing Faculty
5823 Queens Cove
Lisle, IL 60532
(708) 969-3809

## Association of Occupational and Environmental Clinics

The Association of Occupational and Environmental Clinics is dedicated to higher standards of patient-centered, multi-disciplinary care emphasizing prevention and total health through information sharing, quality service and collaborative research. As a national network of clinical facilities, the clinics vary greatly in orientation, physical facilities, and staff capabilities. However, every clinic does offer an on-site staff physician with either board-certification or demonstrated expertise in occupational medicine. Clinics must also have industrial hygienists and other professionals with expertise in occupational and/or environmental health such as nurses, social workers, and health educators either on staff or available through a pre-arranged referral network.

Association of Occupational and Environmental Clinics
1010 Vermont Avenue, #513
Washington, DC 20005
(202) 347-4976

## ALABAMA
Birmingham
Occupational and
Environmental Medicine
Clinic
University of Alabama at
Birmingham
Contact: Timothy J. Key, MD,
MPH
Brian G. Forrester, MD, MPH
(205) 934-7303

## CALIFORNIA
Davis
Occupational and
Environmental Health
Clinic
University of California at
Davis
Contact: Stephen McCurdy,
MD, MPH
Marc Schenker, MD, MPH
(916) 752-3317

Irvine
Occupational and
Environmental Clinic
University of California at
Irvine
Contact: Dean Baker, MD,
MPH
(714) 824-8641

San Francisco
Occupational and
Environmental Medicine
Clinic
University of California at San
Francisco
Contact: Patricia Quinlan,
MPH
Diane Liu, MD, MPH
Jordan Rinker, MD, MPH
(415) 885-7770

## COLORADO
Denver
Occupational and
Environmental Medicine
Division
National Jewish Center for
Immunology and
Respiratory Medicine
Contact: Peggy Mroz, MSPH
Kathleen Kreiss, MD
Cecile Rose, MD, MPH
(303) 398-1520

## CONNECTICUT
Farmington
University of Connecticut
Occupational and
Environmental Medicine
Program
Contact: Eileen Storey, MD,
MPH
(203) 679-2893

New Haven
Yale University Occupational/
Environmental Medicine
Program
Yale School of Medicine
Contact: Mark Cullen, MD,
MPH
(203) 785-5885

Waterbury
Waterbury Occupational
Health
Contact: Gregory McCarthy,
MD, MPH
(203) 573-8114

**DISTRICT OF COLUMBIA**
Washington, DC
  Division of Occupational and
    Environmental Medicine
  George Washington
    University School of
    Medicine
  Contact: Laura Welch, MD,
    MOH
  Rosemary Sokas, MD
  (202) 994-1734

**GEORGIA**
Atlanta
  Environmental and
    Occupational Program
  The Emory Clinic at Perimeter
  Contact: Howard Frumkin,
    MD, DrPH
  Edward Galaid, MD, MPH
  (404) 727-3697
  (404) 248-5478

**ILLINOIS**
Chicago
  Managed Care Occupational
    Health Program
  Mount Sinai Hospital Medical
    Center
  Contact: Gene Miller, Director
  Edward Mogabgab, MD
  (312) 257-6480

  Occupational Medicine Clinic
  Cook County Hospital
  Contact: Stephen Hessl, MD,
    MPH
  (312) 633-5310

University of Illinois
  Occupational Medicine
  Program
  Contact: Linda Forst, MD,
    MS, MPH
  Stephen Hessl, MD, MPH
  (312) 996-1063

**IOWA**
Iowa City
  University of Iowa
    Occupational Medicine
  Clinic
  Department of Internal
    Medicine College of
    Medicine
  Contact: David Schwartz,
    MD, DrPH
  Emma Rosenau, MPH
  (319) 356-8269

**KENTUCKY**
Lexington
  University of Kentucky
    Occupational Medicine
  Program
  Contact: Terence R. Collins,
    MD, MPH
  Chaim Cohen, MD, MPH
(606) 257-5166

**LOUISIANA**
New Orleans
  Ochsner Center for
    Occupational Health
  Contact: Peter G. Casten, MD,
    MPH
  Douglas A. Swift, MD, MSPH
  (504) 838-3955

**MAINE**
Portland
Center for Health Promotion
Contact: Stephen Shannon,
DO, MPH
Sue Upshaw, MD, MPH
(207) 774-7751

**MARYLAND**
Baltimore
Johns Hopkins University
Center for Occupational and
Environmental Health
Contact: Edward J. Bernacki,
MD, MPH
(410) 550-2322

Occupational Health Project
School of Medicine
Division of General Internal
Medicine University of
Maryland
Contact: James Keogh, MD
Julie Gordon, ScM
(410) 706-7464

**MASSACHUSETTS**
Boston
Pulmonary Associates
(Occupational Medicine)
Contact: L. Christine Oliver,
MD, MPH
Elisha Atkins, MD
Dean Hashimoto, MD, JD
David Christiani, MD, MPH
(617) 726-3741

Cambridge
Occupational and
Environmental Health
Center
Cambridge Hospital
Contact: Rose Goldman, MD,
MPH
Susan Rosenwasser, MEd
(617) 498-1580

South Braintree
Center for Occupational and
Environmental Medicine
Massachusetts Respiratory
Hospital
Contact: Diane Plantamura,
MSW
(617) 848-2600

Worcester
Occupational Health Program
Department of Family and
Community Medicine,
University of
Massachusetts
Contact: Glenn Pransky, MD,
Occ.H.
Thomas Hicks, MD, MPH
(508) 856-3093

**MICHIGAN**
Ann Arbor
Occupational Health Program
School of Public Health
University of Michigan
Contact: David Garabrant,
MD, MPH
Tom Robins, MD, MPH
Alfred Franzblau, MD, MPH
(313) 764-2594

Detroit
Division of Occupational
Health
Wayne State University
Department of Family
Medicine
Contact: Raymond Demers,
MD, MPH
Mark Upfal, MD, MPH
James Blessman, MD, MPH
Maryjean Schenk, MD, MPH
Robert Morris, MD, MPH
Sushil Mankani, MD, MPH
(313) 577-1420

East Lansing
Michigan State University
Department of Medicine
Contact: Kenneth Rosenman,
MD, MPH
(517) 353-1846

Lansing
Occupational Health Service
St. Lawrence Hospital and
Health Institute
Contact: R. Michael Kelly,
MD, MPH
(517) 377-0309

Southfield
Center for Occupational and
Environmental Medicine
Contact: Margaret Green,
MD, MPH
Michael Harbut, MD, MPH
(313) 559-6663

**MINNESOTA**
Minneapolis
Columbia Park Medical Group
Occupational Medicine
Department
Contact: Donald Johnson,
MD, MPH
Dorothy Quick, RN, COHN
(612) 572-5710

St. Paul
Ramsey Clinic
Occupational and
Environmental Health and
Occupational Medicine
Residency Training
Contact: Paula Geiger,
Admin. Secretary
William H. Lohman, MD
(612) 221-3771

**NEW JERSEY**
Piscataway
Environmental and
Occupational Health
Clinical Center
Environmental and
Occupational Health
Sciences Institute
UMDNJ-Robert Wood
Johnson Medical School
Contact: Howard Kipen, MD,
MPH
Gail Buckler, RN, MPH,
COHN
(908) 445-0123

**NEW YORK**
Latham
 Eastern NY Occupational
  Health Program
 Contact: Anne Tencza, RN,
  COHN
 Eckhardt Johanning, MD, MSc
 (518) 783-1518

New York
 Bellevue Occupational and
  Environmental Health
  Clinic
 Bellevue Hospital
 Contact: George Friedman-
  Jimenez, MD
 Rafael de la Hoz, MD, MPH
 (212) 561-4572

Mount Sinai
 J. Selikoff Occupational Health
  Clinical Center
 Contact: Stephen Mooser,
  MPH
 Stephen Levin, MD
 Robin Herbert, MD
 (212) 241-6173

Rochester
 Finger Lakes Occupational
  Health Services
 Contact: Julie R. Cataldo,
  Administrator
 (716) 275-1335

Stony Brook
 Center for Occupational and
  Environmental Medicine
 State University of NY School
  of Medicine
 Contact: Wajdy Hailoo, MD,
  MPH
 (516) 444-2167

Syracuse
 Central New York
  Occupational Health
  Clinical Center
 Contact: Michael B. Lax, MD,
  MPH
 (315) 432-8899

**NORTH CAROLINA**
Durham
 Division of Occupational and
  Environmental Medicine
 Duke University Medical
  Center
 Contact: Dennis Darcey, MD,
  MPSH
 Gary Greenberg, MD, MPH
 (919) 286-3232

**OHIO**
Cincinnati
 Center for Occupational
  Health
 Holmes Hospital
 Contact: James Donovan, MD,
  MS
 Douglas Linz, MD, MS
 Susan Pinney, PhD
 (513) 558-1234

 Greater Cincinnati
  Occupational Health
  Center
 Jewish Hospital at Evendale
 Contact: Harriet Applegate,
  Director
 Margaret Atterbury, MD,
  MPH
 (513) 769-0561

Cleveland
Occupational/Environmental
Health Clinic
Department of Family
Medicine
MetroHealth Medical Center
Contact: Kathleen Fagan, MD,
MPH
(216) 778-8087

**OKLAHOMA**
Oklahoma City
University Occupational
Health Sciences
Division of Occupational and
Environmental Medicine
Contact: David Paul, MD,
MPH
Lynn Mitchell, MD, MPH
(405) 271-6177

Tulsa
WorkMed, Inc.
Contact: James W. Small, MD,
MPH
Steve Snyder, MD
Tiari A. Harris, MD, MPH
Lloyd Anderson, MD
(918) 627-4646

**PENNSYLVANIA**
Philadelphia
Occupational Health Service
Department of Community
and Preventive Medicine
Medical College of
Pennsylvania
Contact: Eddy Bresnitz, MD,
MS
Harriet Rubenstein, JD, MPH
(215) 842-6540

Pittsburgh
Occupational and
Environmental Medicine
Program
University of Pittsburgh
Contact: David Tollerud, MD,
MPH
(412) 624-3155

Willow Grove
Center for Occupational and
Environmental Health
Abington Memorial Hospital
Contact: Jessica Herzstein,
MD, MPH
(215) 881-5904

**RHODE ISLAND**
Pawtuckett
Memorial Hospital of Rhode
Island Occupational Health
Service
Brown University
Contact: David G. Kern, MD,
MPH
(401) 729-2859

**TEXAS**
Tyler
Texas Institute of
Occupational Safety and
Health
Contact: Jeffrey Levin, MD,
MSPH
(903) 877-7262

**UTAH**
Salt Lake City
  Rocky Mountain Center for
    Occupational and
    Environmental Health
  Contact:  Anthony Suruda,
    MD, MPH
  Royce Moser, MD, MPH
  (801) 581-5056

**WASHINGTON**
Seattle
  Occupational Medicine
    Program
  University of Washington
  Harborview Medical Center
  Contact:  Scott Barnhart, MD,
    MPH
  Drew Brodkin, MD, MPH
  Matt Keifer, MD, MPH
  (206) 223-3005

**WEST VIRGINIA**
Huntington
  Division of Occupational and
    Environmental Health
  Department of Family and
    Community Medicine
  Marshall University School of
    Medicine
  Contact:  Chris McGuffin, MS
  James Becker, MD
  (304) 696-7045

**CANADA**
Edmonton, Alberta
Occupational Medicine
    Consultation Clinic
  University of Alberta
  Contact:  Linda Cocchiarella,
    MD, MPH
  Tee Guidotti, MD, MPH
  (403) 492-7849

Winnipeg, Manitoba
  MFL Occupational Health
    Centre, Inc.
  Contact:  Judy Cook,
    Executive Director
  (204) 949-0811

## American Organization of Nurse Executives

The American Organization of Nurses Executives (AONE) was established to provide leadership and assistance in the professional development of nursing leaders.  AONE seeks to advance the practice of nursing and patient care through advocacy and research while also playing a vital role in shaping health care public policy at the state and federal levels. AONE also provides educational opportunities for the enhancement of management, leadership, educational, and professional development of nurses as leaders.

American Organization of Nurse Executives
840 N. Lake Shore Drive
Chicago, IL 60611
(312) 280-5213

### Association of Teachers of Preventive Medicine

The Association of Teachers of Preventive Medicine (ATPM) is a national organization for medical educators, practitioners, and students committed to advancing the teaching of all aspects of preventive medicine. The scope of knowledge and competence distinctive to preventive medicine includes biostatistics, epidemiology, administration, environmental and occupational health, the application of social and behavioral factors in health and disease, and primary, secondary, and tertiary prevention measures within clinical medicine. ATPM was founded in 1942 with three basic objectives: (1) advancing medical education; (2) developing instruction, scientific skills and knowledge in preventive medicine; and (3) exchanging experience and ideas among its members.

Association of Teachers of Preventive Medicine
1015 15th Street, N.W.
Suite 405
Washington, DC 20005
(202) 682-1698

### Association of University Environmental Health/Sciences Centers

The Association of University Environmental Health/Sciences Centers (AUEHSC) provides a forum for all of the university-based environmental health science centers supported by the National Institute of Environmental Health. The AUEHSC enables members to exchange information, work in collaboration on projects, and promote cooperation among centers.

Association of University Environmental Health/Science Centers
Mount Sinai School of Medicine
One Gustave L. Levey Place
New York, NY 10029
(212) 241-6173

### Center for Safety in the Arts

The Center for Safety in the Arts (CSA) seeks to gather and disseminate information about health hazards encountered by artists, craftsmen, teachers, children, and others working with art materials. The Center provides on-site assessments of the health and safety features of facilities used by artists, craftsmen, and students; responds to inquiries concerning art-related health hazards; and conducts consultation programs. CSA now offers extensive information through a gopher. To tap into gopher to tmn.com, choose the Arts Wire option, followed by the Center for Safety in the Arts options.

Center for Safety in the Arts
5 Beekman Street
New York, NY 10038
(212) 227-6220

### Committees on Occupational Safety and Health

The Committees on Occupational Safety and Health are non-profit coalitions of local unions and individual workers, physicians, lawyers, and other health safety activists dedicated to the right of each worker to a safe and healthy job. Committees throughout the states provide health and safety training, technical assistance, consultations and on-site evaluations, and contract language assistance.

Committees on Occupational Safety and Health
275 Seventh Avenue
New York, NY 10001
(212) 627-3900

### International Commission on Occupational Health

The International Commission on Occupational Health (ICOH) was founded in 1906 to study new facts in the field of occupational health, to draw the attention of all responsible to the results of study and investigation in occupational health, and to organize meetings on national and international problems in this field. The ICOH has established 26 different scientific committees including a Scientific Committee on Nursing that focus on specific occupational health problems and issues.

International Commission on Occupational Health
Department of Community, Occupational, and Family Medicine
National University Hospital
Lower Kent Ridge Road
0511 Singapore

## International Council of Nurses

The International Council of Nurses (ICN) was founded in 1899 as an multinational nurses' association. The ICN provides a medium through which members can work together in promoting the health of people and the care of the sick across countries. The objectives of ICN are to improve the standards and status of nursing, promote the development of strong national nurses' associations, and serve as the authoritative voice for nurses and the nursing profession worldwide.

International Council of Nurses
1 place Jean-Marteau
CH-12101 Geneva, Switzerland
(22) 731-2960

## MotherRisk Program

The MotherRisk Program will counsel callers about the safety of an exposure to drugs, chemicals, or radiation during pregnancy or breast-feeding. The team of physicians and information specialists gives advice on whether medications, X-rays, or chemicals in the work environment will harm the developing fetus or breast-fed baby.

MotherRisk Program
Hospital for Sick Children
555 University Avenue
Toronto, Ontario, Canada M5G1X8
(416) 813-6780

## National Association of Hispanic Nurses

The National Association of Hispanic Nurses (NAHN) was founded in 1976 for nurses on all educational levels from all Hispanic subgroups and non-Hispanic nurses concerned about the health delivery needs of the Hispanic community and nursing students. NAHN seeks to serve the nursing and health care delivery needs of the Hispanic community and the professional needs of Hispanic nurses. The association also provides forums for Hispanic nurses to analyze, research, and evaluate the health care needs of Hispanic communities and then disseminates findings of that research to local, state, and federal agencies in order to affect policy-making and resource allocation.

National Association of Hispanic Nurses
1501 16th Street, N.W.
Washington, DC 20036
(202) 387-2477

## National Association of School Nurses

The National Association of School Nurses (NASN) is made up of school nurses throughout the country who conduct comprehensive school health programs in public and private schools. The objectives of the NASN are to provide national leadership in the promotion of health services for schoolchildren; to promote school health interests to the nursing and health community and the public; and to monitor legislation pertaining to school nursing. The NASN also provides continuing education programs at the national level and assistance to states for program implementation. NASN also operates the National Board for Certification of School Nurses and certifies school nurses. Besides establishing several workshops and grants for studying children, drug abuse, the female body, and skin care, NASN bestows the annual School Nurse of the Year and Lillian Wald Research Awards.

National Association of School Nurses
Lamplighter Lane
P.O. Box 1300
Scarborough, ME 04070
(207) 883-2117

## National Black Nurses Association

The National Black Nurses Association (NBNA) functions as a professional support group and as an advocacy group for the black community and their health care. NBNA recruits and assists blacks interested in pursing nursing as a career and presents scholarships to student nurses who have excelled in the field.

National Black Nurses Association
1012 10th Street N.W.
Washington, DC 20001-4492
(202) 393-6870

## National Council of State Boards of Nursing

The National Council of State Boards of Nursing (NCSBN) was founded in 1978 as the national council for all state boards of nursing. The NCSBN seeks to assist member boards in administrating the National Council Licensure Examinations for Registered Nurses and Practical Nurses and works to insure relevancy of the exams to current nursing practice. The council also aids individual boards in the collection and analysis of information pertaining to the licensure and discipline of nurses. The NCSBN also provides consultative services, conducts research, and sponsors educational programs.

National Council of State Boards of Nursing
676 N. St. Clair, Suite 550
Chicago, IL 60611
(312) 787-6555

## National Environmental Health Association

The National Environmental Health Association (NEHA) is a professional society of persons engaged in environmental health and protection for governmental agencies, public health and environmental protection agencies, industry, colleges, and universities. NEHA also conducts national professional registration programs and offers continuing education opportunities for interested professionals.

National Environmental Health Association
720 S. Colorado Blvd.
Suite 970, S. Tower
Denver, CO 80222
(301) 756-9090

## National League for Nursing

The National League for Nursing (NLN) was established in 1952 for individuals and leaders in nursing and other health professions interested in solving health care problems. The NLN works to assess nursing needs, improve organized nursing services and nursing education, foster collaboration between nursing and other health and community services, provide tests used in the selection of applicants to schools of nursing, and prepare tests used in evaluating nursing student progress and nursing service test. On a national level, the NLN accredits nursing education programs and community health agencies while collecting and disseminating data on nursing services and education.

National League for Nursing
350 Hudson Street
New York, NY 10014
(800) 669-1656

## National Student Nurses' Association

The National Student Nurses' Association (NSNA) comprises students currently enrolled in state-approved nursing schools for the preparation of becoming registered nurses. NSNA seeks to aid in the development of the individual nursing student and urges students, as future health professionals, to be aware of and to contribute to improving the health care of all people. NSNA also encourages programs and activities in state groups concerning nursing, health, and the community.

National Student Nurses' Association
555 W. 57th Street
Suite 1327
New York, NY 10019
(212) 581-2211

## Nurses Educational Funds

The Nurses Educational Funds (NEF) seeks to establish, maintain, and administer funds to provide financial assistance to registered nurses studying for advanced degrees. The NEF also helps formulate policies for the administration of such funds while collecting and managing all funds contributed to it.

Nurses Educational Funds
555 W. 57th Street, 13th Floor
New York, NY 10019
(212) 582-8820

## Pesticide Education Center

Founded in 1933 to educate the public about the hazards and health effects of pesticides, the Pesticide Education Center works with community groups, workers, individuals, and others harmed by or concerned about risks to their health from exposure to pesticides used in agriculture, the home and garden, and other environmental and industrial uses. Its goal is to provide critical information about pesticides so that the public can make more informed decisions and choices. The PEC provides information, curricular materials, and help with seminars and workshops on a nationwide basis.

Pesticide Education Center
P.O. Box 420870
San Francisco, CA 94142-0870
(415) 391-8511

## Sigma Theta Tau International

Sigma Theta Tau International (STTI) was founded in 1822 as a honorary society for nurses. STTI provides members with the opportunity to access information through their libraries, references, and databases, while also recognizing excellence in the field of nursing with awards and grants for research. STTI seeks to promote the profession of nursing as leaders, advocates, and pertinent players in the care of the individual and community's health.

Sigma Theta Tau International
550 W. North Street
Indianapolis, IN 46202
(317) 634-8171

## Society for Occupational and Environmental Health

The Society for Occupational and Environmental Health (SOEH) includes scientists, academicians, and industry and labor representatives who seek to improve the quality of both working and living places by operating as a neutral forum for conferences involving all aspects of occupational and environmental health. SOEH's activities include studying specific categories of hazards, as well as developing methods for assessment of health effects and diseases associated with particular jobs.

Society for Occupational and Environmental Health
6728 Old McLean Village Drive
McLean, VA 22101
(703) 556-9222

## Teratogen Exposure Registry and Surveillance

The Teratogen Exposure Registry and Surveillance (TERAS) is a network of geneticists and pathologists studying human embryos and fetuses exposed to teratogens. TERAS maintains information networks for consultation and evaluations.

Teratogen Exposure Registry and Surveillance
Department of Pathology
Brigham and Women's Hospital
75 Francis Street
Boston, MA
(617) 732-6507

## WorldWatch Institute

The WorldWatch Institute is a research organization that aims to encourage a reflective and deliberate approach to global problem-solving. The Institute seeks to anticipate global problems and social trends and to focus attention on emerging global issues, including population growth, family planning, environmental degradation, and renewable energy options.

WorldWatch Institute
1776 Massachusetts Avenue, N.W.
Washington, DC 20036
(202) 452-1999

## SELECTED TOPICAL RESOURCES

*AIR POLLUTION*
American Lung Association
  (212) 315-8700
EPA Clean Air Act
  (202) 382-7548

*ART SUPPLIES*
Center for Safety in the Arts
(212) 277-6220

*ASBESTOS*
EPA Asbestos Programs
  (800) 368-5888

*CANCER INFORMATION*
National Cancer Institute
  (800) 4-CANCER
EPA Carcinogen Assessment
  Group
  (202) 382-5898

CHEMICAL EMERGENCIES
Chemical Spills Emergency
    Hotline
    (800) 535-0202
EPA Hazardous Waste Hotline
    (800) 535-0202
ATSDR Emergency Hotline
    (404) 639-6300

CONSUMER PRODUCT SAFETY
Consumer Product Safety
    Commission
    (800) 638-2772

HAZARDOUS WASTE
EPA Emergency Planning and
    Community Right to Know
    Hotline
    (800) 535-0202
Integrated Risk Information
    System (IRIS)
    (202) 475-6743
IRIS User Support
    (513) 569-7254
Superfund Records of Decision
    (703) 920-9810
State Health Departments

LEAD
National Center for
    Environmental Health (CDC)
    (404) 488-4880
National Lead Information Center
    (800) LEAD-FYI
Child and Maternal Health
    Clearinghouse
    (202) 625-8410

LUNG DISEASE
American Lung Association
    (212) 315-8700
LUNGLINE/National Jewish
    Hospital
    (800) 222-5864

OCCUPATIONAL HEALTH
National Institute for
    Occupational Safety and
    Health
    (800) 356-4674
Occupational Safety and Health
    Administration
    (202) 219-8151

PESTICIDES
EPA National Pesticides Hotline
    (800) 535-PEST
National Pesticide
    Telecommunications Network
    (800) 858-7378

POISONING
Poison Control Centers

PREGNANCY CONCERNS
MotherRisk Program
    (416) 813-7378

RADON
EPA Office of Radon Programs
    (202) 475-9605
National Radon Hotline
    (800) SOS-RADON
State Health Departments

SMOKE
American Lung Association
    (212) 315-8700

*TOXIC SUBSTANCES*
American Chemical Society's
 Chemical Referral Center
 (202) 887-1315
ATSDR Emergency Response
 Branch
 (404) 639-6300
ATSDR Toxicological Profiles
 (404) 639-6000

EPA Toxic Substances Control Act
 (TSCA)
 Information Line
 (202) 554-1404
EPA Toxic Chemical Release
 Inventory System
 (800) 535-0202

*WATER*
EPA Safe Drinking Water Hotline
 (800) 426-4791

## COMPUTERIZED INFORMATION SERVICES

Computerized information services have become a valuable link in providing users with up-to-date information, resources, and opportunities for interaction with others interested in similar topics. The following list is by no means comprehensive, but merely provides points of access to relevant information and communication list-servers.

### Internet

*Department of Energy's Environment, Safety, and Health Technical Information Service*

In 1993, DOE released its new computer-based information service, called the Environment, Safety, and Health Technical Information Service (TIS). TIS is designed to provide the DOE community with technical information that is reliable, current, and easy to use. Eventually, TIS will replace the current Safety Performance Measurement System (SPMS). For more information, please address any questions to the TIS Helpline at (208) 526-8955 or send e-mail to support@tis.inel.gov.

*Electronic Green Journal*

The ELECTRONIC GREEN JOURNAL is a professional refereed publication from the University of Idaho devoted to disseminating information concerning sources of international environmental topics including: assessment, conservation, development, disposal, education, hazards, pollution, resources, technology, and treatment. The journal serves communities as an educational environmental resource, and includes both practical and scholarly articles, bibliographies, reviews, editorial comments, and announcements. The journal is currently available via gopher, world-wide web, or ftp. Subscriptions are being planned for the future. To tap into the journal through gopher, type gopher.uidaho.edu and choose University of Idaho Electronic Publications; to tap in through World-Wide Web (WWW) type http://gopher.uidaho.edu/ 1/UI_gopher/library/egj/; or to tap in through ftp, type ftp.uidaho.edu.

## EnviroLink Network

The Envirolink Network is a non-profit organization that is dedicated to facilitating communication on environmental issues. The network is composed of over 400,000 people in 93 countries. The Network has recently created a new network entitled EnviroFreenet. EnviroFreenet offers e-mail accounts, environmental billboards, chat conferences, the EnviroGopher, the EnviroWeb, and access to almost every other Internet Service available. The network can be accessed using either telnet or gopher. EnviroFreenet can be reached through telnet with the address envirolink.org. Directions then follow. If you have access to gopher, go to the main gopher list and choose international organizations and then choose "EnviroGopher," followed by "Connect to EnviroFreenet" or gopher to: envirolink.org port 70.

## HazDat

The HazDat system is a scientific and administrative database developed by ATSDR to provide rapid access to information on the release of hazardous substances from Superfund sites or from emergency events and on the effects of these substances on the health of human populations. The source documents used for the initial development of HazDat include environmental and health data contained in Agency products and in other non-Agency site characterization documents as appropriate. ATSDR's products include health assessments and supporting documentation for over 1,200 sites, toxicological profiles for over 150 substances, and more than 2,000 health consultations. ATSDR staff enter data into HazDat on a continuing basis. HazDat is available to the public over the Internet through a World-Wide Web (WWW) server. Access can be gained through: http://atsdr1.atsdr.cdc.gov:8080/atsdrhome.html.

## Medical List—A Guide to On Line Medical Resources

The Medical List provides a complete listing of Internet resources connected with health, disease, therapy, and clinical medicine. This resource list is offered in text form as The Medical List and as Medical

Matrix—a hypertest database accessible using World Wide Web browsers like Mosaic. The Medical List is the text of Healthmatrix—a Windows Help, icon drive, hypertext presentation of the database. For more information, call (209) 466-6878.

Gopher access to The Medical List is available at the URL:(Uniform Resource Locator)gopher://una.hh.lib.umich.edu:70/11/inetdirs/sciences/medclin:malet. Gopher allows key word searching and e-mail of this document to any Internet address. Access can also be gained through ftp—frp2.cc.ukans.edu pub/hmatrix/ and get file medlst94.txt or medlst94.zip.

Medical Matrix is a project of the Internet Working Group of the American Medical Informatics Association. Medical Matrix uses icons and keyword searches to locate on line medical resources. Access can be gained through: http://kuhttp.cc.ukans.edu/cwis/units/medcntr/Lee/HOMEPAHE.HTML.

## Nightingale

Nightingale is a gopher server dedicated to providing the nursing community with easy access to information which is unique or pertinent to the nursing profession. Resources and information is available on topics such as research, practice, education, professional nursing communications, publications, and other nursing resources. Access can be gained through: http://nightingale.con.utk.edu./00/homepage.html.

## Nursing Institutes on Internet

Arizona Health Sciences Center—College of Nursing (http://www.medlib.arizona.edu)
Brigham Young University—College of Nursing (http://nurse.byu.edu)
Duke University Nursing Services (http://nursing-www.mc.duke.edu/nursing/nshomepg.htm)
East Tennessee State University—College of Nursing (http://www.east-tenn-st.edu/~etsucon)
European Summerschool of Nursing Informatics (http://care4all.nursing.nl:8080/sumsch/sumhome.html)
Ohio State University—College of Nursing (http://www.con.ohio-state.edu/index.htm)
University of California at San Francisco—School of Nursing (http://nurseweb.ucsf.edu/www/ucsfson.htm)
University of Central Florida—School of Nursing (http://pegasus.cc.usf.edu/~wink/nursing.department.html)

University of Delaware—College of Nursing (http://www.udel.edu./
brentt/UD_Nursing.html)
University of New Hampshire (http://pubpages.unh.edu/~tpcox/
nsg.html)
University of Iowa—College of Nursing (http://
coninfor.nursing.uiowa.edu/index.htm)
University of Louisville, Kentucky (http://www.louisville.edu)
University of Maryland—College of Nursing (http://
www.nursing.ab.umd.edu)
University of Missouri, Columbia (http://www.missouri.edu/
~nurswalk/nmwhome.html)
University of Pennsylvania—School of Nursing (http://
dolphin.upenn.edu/~nursing)
University of Tennessee, Knoxville—Nursing Gopher (http://
nightingale.con.utk.edu:70/01homepage.html)
University of Washington—School of Nursing (http://
www.son.hs.washington.edu)
West Virginia University—School of Nursing (http://
www.hsc.wvu.edu/son/index.htm)

## Nursing Internet Resources

The Nursing Internet Resources provides a guide and link to nursing
resources on-line.  Access can be gained through:
http://www.csv.warwick.ac.uk:8000/nurse-resources.html
or gopher-p1papers/nurse.csv.warwick.ac.uk

## Nursing Network Forum

The Nursing Network Forum is operated and managed by Mid-At-
lantic Network Associates, Inc. as a resource and discussion forum for
nurses around the country.  Services on the Nursing Network Forum
include (1) a message base for discussion of various aspects of nursing,
career opportunities, and nursing school experiences; (2) a conferencing
area where users talk "live" with other nurses; (3) a library area filled
with resources and on-line continuing education programs provided
through the University of Maryland and accredited by ANCCCA (these
programs can be completed in the home while earning accredited contact
hours toward continuing education units); and (4) a direct nursing gopher and usernet discussion group access.  Although the forum is not
free, trial periods are provided.

For additional information, please contact the Nursing Network Forum at (800) 695-4002 or through internet at nurse@delphi.com or nurse@clark.net.

## WHO Global Environmental Epidemiology Network, GEENET

The Network was established in 1987 as a means for the World Health Organization to strengthen education, training, and research in institutions involved in epidemiological teaching and research on the health effects of environmental hazards, and other epidemiological applications in environmental and occupational health.

The Network aims at improved communication and collaboration between institutions in this field in developed and developing countries. A series of documents with information of value for training and research development is prepared for the Network and lists of Network members are distributed on a regular basis. Training and research promotion workshops are organized in collaboration with national and international agencies.

For more information, write: WHO GEENET, Environmental Epidemiology, World Health Organization, 1211 Geneva, Switzerland.

## List Servers

### Air Pollution and Biology

The address is mailbase@mailbase.ac.uk; and you can join by sending the message join airpollution-biology Firstname Lastname and your address.

### EHS-L Environmental Health Systems

The address is listserv@ALBNYDH2; and you can join by sending the message subscribe EHS-L Firstname Lastname and your address.

### ENVBEH-L Environment and Human Behavior

The address is listserv@POLYVM; and you can join by sending the message subscribe ENVBEH-L Firstname Lastname and your address.

### Enviroethics

The address is mailbase@mailbase.ac.uk; and you can join by sending the message join enviroethics Firstname Lastname and your address.

*NURSENET*

NURSENET provides discussion about pertinent nursing issues facing the profession. To subscribe send your Firstname Lastname to listserv@vm.utcc.utoronto.ca sub nursenet.

*NURSERES Nurses Research List*

NURSERES allows discussion of research being conducted in the field of nursing. To join send your Firstname Lastname to listserv@kentvm.kent.edu with a message of SUB NURSERES.

*NRSINGED Nursing Educators List*

NRSINGED is a discussion group of nursing educators concerning the various issues and aspects of nursing education. To join send your Firstname Lastname with the message SUB NRSINGED to listserv@ulkyvm.louisville.edu.

*Occup-Env Med List (Occupational and Environmental Medicine Listing on Internet)*

Occupational and environmental medicine represents a growing clinical and public health discipline, seeking to evaluate and prevent the diseases and health effects that may be related to exposures at work and from other environments. The Occup-Env Med Mail-list provides a moderated forum for announcements, dissemination of text files and academic discussion. The forum is designed to allow presentation of clinical vignettes, synopses of new regulatory issues and reports of interesting items from publication elsewhere (both the medical and the non-medical journals).

To subscribe, send a message of: subscribe occ-env-med-l "first name last name" to occ-env-med-l@mc.duke.edu.

To post a message send the message to: occ-env-med-l@duke.edu

*SNURSE-L*

SNURSE-L is a list server for undergraduate nursing students. To join send mail to listserv@ubvm.cc.buffalo.edu with the message SUB SNURSE-L Firstname Lastname.

## Other Gophers/Internet Relevant to
## Environmental Health and Nursing

*Division of Environmental Health and Safety*

  gopher://romulus.ehs.uiuc.edu:70/11

*The Environmental Magazine*

  gopher://gopher.internet.com:2100/11/collected/d

*NCLEX Nursing Careers*

  http://www.kaplan.com/etc/nclex_index.html

*National Institute of Environmental Health Sciences (NIEHS)*

  gopher://gopher.niehs.nih.gov/1

*NURSE at Warwick University*

  gopher://gopher.nurse.csv.warwick.ac.uk
  http://www.csv.warwick.ac.uk:8000/

*U.S. Environmental Protection Agency*

  gopher://gopher.rtpnc.epa.gov/1

### Computer-Based Databases*

  The National Library of Medicine (NLM) is the world's largest research library in a single scientific or professional field. The library collects materials in all major areas of the health sciences, as well as in such areas as chemistry, physics, botany, and zoology.

  The Library's computer-based Medical Literature Analysis and Retrieval System (MEDLARS) and toxicology (TOXLINE) databases provide on-line bibliographic access to the Library's store of biomedical information. For information about access to MEDLARS and TOXLINE services, contact: MEDLARS Management Section, National Library of Medicine, 8600 Rockville Pike, Bethesda, MD 20894, (301) 496-1131, (800) 638-8480 (outside Maryland).

---

*Adapted from Murdock, BS, ed. 1991. *Environmental Issues in Primary Care*. Minnesota: Minnesota Department of Health.

Primary biomedical data bases included on the MEDLARS system are:

**MEDLINE** indexes articles from over 3200 biomedical journals published in the United States and abroad. MEDLINE is indexed using NLM's controlled vocabulary, MESH (Medical Subject Headings), and contains all citations indexed in INDEX MEDICUS. Produced by the National Library of Medicine.

**TOXLINE** is designed to offer comprehensive bibliographic coverage of toxicological information. It covers the pharmacological, biochemical, physiological, environmental, and toxicological effects of chemicals and drugs. Produced by Specialized Information Services of the National Library of Medicine.

**TOXNET (Toxicology Data Network)** is a computerized system of toxicological data banks operated by the National Library of Medicine, and is part of the broader MEDLARS system.

The TOXNET software consists of modules to build, edit, and review the records of constituent data banks.

**CCRIS (Chemical Carcinogenesis Research Information System)** is a factual data bank sponsored by the National Cancer Institute. It contains data derived from both short- and long-term bioassays on approximately 1200 chemicals.

**ETICBACK (Environmental Teratology Information Center Backfile)** is a bibliographic data base covering teratology and development toxicology.

**TRI (Toxic Chemical Release Inventory)** contains information on the annual estimated releases of toxic chemicals to the environment in the United States. These data include the names and addresses of the facilities and the amounts of certain toxic chemicals they release to the air, water, or land or transfer to waste sites.

**HSDB (Hazardous Substances Data Bank)** is a comprehensive data base containing records for over 4100 toxic or potentially toxic chemicals. It contains information in such areas as toxicity, environmental fate, human exposure, chemical safety, waste disposal, emergency handling, and regulatory requirements.

**IRIS (Integrated Risk Information System)** is an on-line data base built by the Environmental Protection Agency (EPA). It contains EPA carcinogenic and noncarcinogenic health risk and regulatory information on about 400 chemicals. For more information, call (513) 569-7254.

**RTECS (Registry of Toxic Effects of Chemical Substances)** contains toxic effects data for approximately 100,000 chemicals. It is built and maintained by the National Institute for Occupational Safety and Health (NIOSH). Acute and chronic effects are covered in such areas as skin/eye irritation, carcinogenicity, mutagenicity, and reproductive consequences. Contact: (800) 35-NIOSH

**DIRLINE (NLM's Directory of Information Resources on-line)** is an on-line database containing information on approximately 15,000 organizations that provide information and services directly to requesters. DIRLINE is available on-line through the MEDLARS system and can also be searched with GRATEFUL MED software. Contact: (301) 496-1131

**Various software packages are available for access to MEDLARS, including:**

**GRATEFUL MED**, a microcomputer software interface that assists users in performing on-line searches of NLM's databases. GRATEFUL MED can be bought from the National Technical Information Service (NTIS).

**CHEMLEARN** (NTIS), an interactive, microcomputer-based training package for CHEMLINE. Produced by Specialized Information Services of the National Library of Medicine, it runs on IBM-PC/XT/AT/PS/2 compatibles. CHEMLEARN is available from NTIS, product number PB88-218144. For more information on the contents of the software, call (301) 496-1131.

**TOXLEARN** is an interactive, microcomputer-based training package for TOXLINE. Its menu-driven structure allows users to make choices in learning about basic aspects of TOXLINE. It contains approximately four hours of interactive instruction and is produced by the Specialized Information Services of the National Library of Medicine. TOXLEARN runs on IBM-PC compatibles and is available from NTIS, product number PB88-155766. For more information on the contents of the software, call (301) 496-1131.

## GENERAL REFERENCES

Aldrich, T., and Griffith, J. 1993. *Environmental Epidemiology and Risk Assessment*. New York: Van Nostrand Reinhold.

Anderson, E.T., and McFarlane, J.M. 1995. *Community as Partner: Theory and Practice of Nursing*. Philadelphia: J.B. Lippincott.

Bullough, B., and Bullough, V. 1990. *Nursing in the Community*. St. Louis: C.V. Mosby.

Burgess, W.A. 1981. *Recognition of Health Hazards in Industry: A Review of Materials and Processes*. New York: John Wiley and Sons.

California Public Health Foundation. 1992. *Kids and the Environment: Toxic Hazards*. Berkeley: California Public Health Foundation.

Chivian, E., McCally, M., Hu, H., and Haines, A., eds. 1993. *Critical Condition: Human Health and the Environment*. Cambridge: MIT Press.

Clemen-Stone, S., Eigsti, D.G., and McGuire, S.L. 1995. *Comprehensive Family and Community Health Nursing*. 4th ed. St. Louis: C.V. Mosby.

Davis, A.J., and Aroskar, M.A. 1991. *Ethical Dilemmas in Nursing Practice*. 3rd ed. Norwalk, CT: Appleton and Lange.

Gary, F., and Kavanagh, C.T. 1991. *Psychiatric Mental Health Nursing*. Philadelphia: J.B. Lippincott.

Girdando, D.A. 1986. *Occupational Health Promotion: A Practical Guide to Program Development*. New York: MacMillian Publishing Co.

Gorall, A.H., May, L.A., and Mulley, A.G. 1995. *Primary Care Medicine*. 3rd ed. Philadelphia: J.B. Lippincott.

Green, L.W. 1990. *Community Health*. 6th ed. St. Louis: Times Mirror/Mosby.

Guidotti, T.L. 1989. *Occupational Health Services: A Practical Approach*. Chicago: American Medical Association.

Hansen, D.F., ed. 1991. *The Work Environment*. Chelsea, MI: Lews Publishers, Inc.

Hersey, P., and Blanchard, K. 1993. *Management of Organizationl Behavioral: Utilizing Human Resources*. Englewood Cliffs, NJ: Prentice-Hall.

Institute of Medicine (IOM). 1993. *Indoor Allergens: Assessing and Controlling Adverse Health Effects*. Washington, DC: National Academy Press.

IOM. 1995. *Environmental Medicine: Integrating a Missing Element into Medical Education*. Washington, DC: National Academy Press.

International Labour Office (ILO). 1983. *Encyclopedia of Occupational Health and Safety*. 3rd ed., 2 volumes. Geneva: ILO.

Kornberg, J.P. 1992. *The Workplace Walkthrough* (Vol. 1). Boca Raton, FL: Lewis Publishers.

LaDou, J. 1990. *Occupational Medicine*. Norwalk, CT: Appleton and Lange.

Last, J.M., and Wallace, R.B., eds. 1992. *Public Health and Human Ecology*. Norwalk: Appleton and Lange.

Levy, B., and Wegman, D. 1995. *Occupational Health: Recognizing and Preventing Work-related Disease*. 3rd ed. Boston: Little, Brown.

Lindberg, J.B., Hunter, M.L., and Kruszewski, A.Z. 1994. *Introduction to Nursing: Concepts, Issues and Opportunities*. 2nd ed. Philadelphia: J.B. Lippincott.

Lybarger, J.A., Spengler, R.F., and DeRosa, C.T. 1993. *Priority Health Conditions*. Washington, DC: ATSDR.

Marquis, B.L., and Huston, C.J. 1992. *Leadership Roles and Management Functions in Nursing*. Philadelphia: J.B. Lippincott.

Mason, D.J., Talbott, S.W., and Leavitt, J.K. 1993. *Policy and Politics for Nurses: Action and Change in the Workplace, Government, Organizations, and Community*. 2nd ed. Philadelphia: W.B. Saunders.

McCunney, R.J., ed. 1994. *A Practical Approach to Occupational and Environmental Medicine.* Boston: Little, Brown.

McLaughlin, F.E., and Marasuilo, L.A. 1990. *Advanced Nursing and Health Care Research.* Philadelphia: W.B. Saunders.

Murdock, B.S. 1991. *Environmental Issues in Primary Care.* Minneapolis: Freshwater Foundation's Health and the Environment Digest.

Murray, R.B., and Zentner, J.P. 1989. *Nursing Assessment and Health Promotion: Strategies Through the Life Span.* 4th ed. Norwalk, CT: Appleton & Lange.

National Library of Medicine. 1989. *Improving Health Professionals' Access to Information: Challenges and Opportunities for the National Library of Medicine.* Washington, DC: National Library of Medicine.

National Research Council (NRC). 1989. *Improving Risk Communication.* Washington, DC: National Academy Press.

NRC. 1991. *Environmental Epidemiology.* Washington, DC: National Academy Press.

Paul, M., ed. 1993. *Occupational and Environmental Reproductive Hazards: A Guide for Clinicians.* Baltimore, MD: Williams and Wilkins.

Polit, D.F., and Hungler, B.P. 1995. *Nursing Research: Principles and Methods.* 5th ed. Philadelphia: J.B. Lippincott.

Rogers, B. 1994. *Occupational Health Nursing: Concepts and Practice.* Philadelphia: W.B. Saunders.

Rogers, B., Mastroianni, K., and Randolph, S.A. 1992. *Occupational Health Nursing Guidelines: Primary Clinical Conditions.* Boston: OEM Press.

Rom, W, ed. 1992. *Environmental and Occupational Medicine, Second Edition.* Boston: Little, Brown.

Rosenstock, L., and Cullen, M. 1986. *Clinical Occupational Medicine.* Philadelphia: W.B. Saunders.

Rosenstock, L., and Cullen, M. 1994. *Textbook of Clinical Occupational and Environmental Medicine.* Philadelphia: W.B. Saunders.

Sandman, P., Chess, C., and Hance, B.J. 1991. *Improving Dialogue with Communities: A Risk Communication Manual for Government.* New Brunswick: Rutgers University and New Jersey Department of Environmental Protection and Energy.

Saucier, K.A. 1991. *Perspectives on Family and Community Health.* St. Louis: C.V. Mosby.

Silbergeld, E.K. 1993. *Investing in Prevention: Opportunities to Reduce Disease and Health Care Costs Through Identifying and Reducing Environmental Contributions to Preventable Disease.* Washington, DC: Environmental Defense Fund.

Smith, C.M., and Maure, F.A. 1995. *Community Health Nursing: Theory and Practice.* Philadelphia: W.B. Saunders.

Stanhope, M., and Lancaster, J. 1992. *Community Health Nursing: Process and Practice for Promoting Health.* 3rd ed. St. Louis: C.V. Mosby.

Stritter, F.T. 1992. Faculty Evaluation and Development. *Handbook of Health Professionals Education* 13:294–318.

Sullivan, J.B., and Krieger, G.R. 1992. *Hazardous Materials Toxicology: Clinical Principles in Environmental Health.* Baltimore: Williams and Wilkins.

Tarcher, AB, ed. 1992. *Principles and Practice of Environmental Medicine.* New York: Plenum Medical Book Co.

Upton, A.C., and Graber, E. 1993. *Staying Healthy in a Risky Environment: The New York University Medical Center Family Guide.* New York: Simon and Schuster.

U.S. Environmental Protection Agency. 1988a. *Proposed Guidelines for Assessing Female Reproductive Risk. Federal Register* 53:24834–24847.

U.S. Environmental Protection Agency. 1988b. *Proposed Guidelines for Assessing Male Reproductive Risk. Federal Register* 53:24850–24869.

U.S. Environmental Protection Agency. 1992. *Guidelines for Exposure Assessment. Federal Register* 57:22888–22938.

Waltz, C., Strickland, O.L., and Lenz, E. 1991. *Measurement in Nursing Research.* 2nd ed. Philadelphia: F.A. Davis.

Weeks, J. 1991. *Preventing Occupational Disease and Injury.* Washington, DC: American Public Health Association.

Wilkinson, J.M. 1992. *Nursing Process in Action.* Redwood City, CA: Addison Wesley.

Williams, P.L., and Burson, J.L. 1985. *Industrial Toxicology: Safety and Health Applications in the Workplace.* New York: Van Nostrand Reinhold.

Wold, S.J. 1990. *Community Health Nursing: Issues and Topics.* Norwalk, CT: Appleton and Lange.

World Health Organization: Our Planet, Our Health. 1992. *Report of the WHO Commission on Health and Environment.* Geneva: World Health Organization.

# Tables of Environmental Agents and Health Effects, Work-Related Diseases and Conditions, and Selected Job Categories and Associated Diseases and Conditions

TABLE D-l: Environmental Agents, Their Sources and Potential
Exposures, and Adverse Health Effects: Metals and Metallic Compounds,
Hydrocarbons, Irritant Gases, Chemical Asphyxiates, and Pesticides

| Agent | Exposure | Route of Entry | Systems(s) Affected |
|-------|----------|----------------|---------------------|
| **Metals and Metallic Compounds** | | | |
| Arsenic | Alloyed with lead and copper for hardness; manufacturing of pigments, glass, pharmaceuticals; byproduct in copper smelting; insecticides; fungicides; rodenticides; tanning | Inhalation and ingestion of dust and fumes | Neuromuscular Gastrointestinal Skin Pulmonary |
| Arsine | Accidental byproduct of reaction of arsenic with acid; used in semi-conductor industry | Inhalation of gas | Hematopoietic |
| Beryllium | Hardening agent in metal alloys; special use in nuclear energy production; metal refining or recovery | Inhalation of fumes or dust | Pulmonary (and other systems) |
| Cadmium | Electroplating; solder for aluminum; metal alloys, process engraving; nickel-cadmium batteries | Inhalation or ingestion of fumes or dust | Pulmonary Renal |
| Chromium | In stainless and heat-resistant steel and alloy steel; metal plating; chemical and pigment manufacturing; photography | Percutaneous absorption, inhalation, ingestion | Pulmonary Skin |

| Primary Manifestations | Aids in Diagnosis[a] | Remarks |
|---|---|---|
| Peripheral neuropathy, sensory-motor<br>Nausea and vomiting, diarrhea, constipation<br>Dermatitis, finger and toenail striations, skin cancer, nasal septum perforation<br>Lung cancer | Arsenic in urine | |
| Intravascular hemolysis: hemoglobinuria, jaundice, oliguria or anuria | Arsenic in urine | |
| Granulomatosis and fibrosis | Beryllium in urine (acute); Beryllium m tissue (chronic); chest x ray; immunologic tests (such as lymphocyte transformation) may also be useful | Pulmonary changes virtually indistinguishable from sarcoid on chest x ray |
| Pulmonary edema (acute); Emphysema (chronic)<br>Nephrosis | Urinary protein | Also a respiratory tract carcinogen |
| Lung cancer<br>Dermatitis, skin ulcers, nasal septum perforation | Urinary chromate (questionable value) | |

continued on next page

TABLE D-l: Continued

| Agent | Exposure | Route of Entry | Systems(s) Affected |
|---|---|---|---|
| Lead | Storage batteries; manufacturing of paint, enamel, ink, glass, rubber ceramics, chemical industry | Ingestion of dust, inhalation of dust or fumes | Hematologic Renal Gastrointestinal Neuromuscular CNS Reproductive |
| Mercury (Elemental) | Electronic equipment; paint; metal and textile production; catalyst in chemical manufacturing; pharmaceutical production | Inhalation of vapor; slight percutaneous absorption | Pulmonary CNS |
| (Inorganic) | | Some inhalation and GI and percutaneous absorption | Pulmonary Renal CNS |
| (Organic) | Agricultural and industrial poisons | Efficient GI absorption, percutaneous absorption, and inhalation | Skin CNS |

| Primary Manifestations | Aids in Diagnosis[a] | Remarks |
|---|---|---|
| Anemia<br>Nephropathy<br>Abdominal pain ("colic")<br>Palsy ("wrist drop")<br>Encephalopathy, behavioral abnormalities<br>Spontaneous abortions (?) | Blood lead<br>Urinary ALA<br>Zinc proto-porphyrin (ZPP); free erythrocyte protophyrin (FEP) | Lead toxicity, unlike that of mercury, is believed to be reversible, with the exception of late renal and some CNS effects. |
| Acute pneumonitis; Neuro-psychiatric changes (erethism); tremor | Urinary mercury | Mercury illustrates several principles. The chemical form has a profound effect on its toxicology, as is the case for many metals. Effects of mercury are highly variable. Though inorganic mercury poisoning is primarily renal, elemental and organic poisoning are primarily neurological. The responses are difficult to quantify, so dose-response data are generally unavailable. Classic tetrad of gingivitis, sialorrhea, irritability, and tremor is associated with both elemental and inorganic mercury poisoning; the four signs are not generally seen together. Many effects of mercury toxicity, especially those in CNS, are irreversible. |
| Acute pneumonitis<br>Proteinuria<br>Variable | Urinary mercury | |
| Dermatitis<br>Sensorimotor changes, visual field constriction, tremor | Blood and urine mercury, but ? sensitivity | |

continued on next page

TABLE D-l: Continued

| Agent | Exposure | Route of Entry | Systems(s) Affected |
|---|---|---|---|
| Nickel | Corrosion-resistant alloys; electroplating; catalyst production; nickel-cadmium batteries | Inhalation of dust or fumes | Skin<br><br>Pulmonary |
| Zinc oxide[b] | Welding byproduct; rubber manufacturing | Inhalation of dust or fumes that are freshly generated | |

### Hydrocarbons

| Agent | Exposure | Route of Entry | Systems(s) Affected |
|---|---|---|---|
| Benzene | Manufacturing of organic chemicals, detergents, pesticides, solvents, paint removers; used as a solvent | Inhalation of vapor; slight percutaneous absorption | CNS<br>Hematopoietic<br>Skin |
| Toluene | Organic chemical manufacturing; solvent; fuel component | Inhalation of vapor, percutaneous absorption of liquid | CNS<br><br><br>Skin |
| Xylene | A wide variety of uses as a solvent; an ingredient of paints, lacquers, varnishes, inks, dyes, adhesives, cements; an intermediate in chemical manufacturing | Inhalation of vapor; slight percutaneous absorption of liquid | Pulmonary<br><br>Eyes, nose, throat<br>CNS |
| Ketones (Acetone) (Methylethyl ketone—MEK) (Methyl n-propyl ketone—MPK) (Methyl n-butyl ketone—MBK) (Methyl iso-butyl ketone—MIBK) | A wide variety of uses as solvents and intermediates in chemical manufacturing | Inhalation of vapor, percutaneous absorption of liquid | CNS<br>PNS<br><br>Skin |

| Primary Manifestations | Aids in Diagnosis[a] | Remarks |
|---|---|---|
| Sensitization dermatitis ("nickel itch") Lung and paranasal sinus cancer | | |
| "Metal fume fever" (fever, chills, and other symptoms) | Urinary zinc (useful as an indicator of with exposure, not for acute diagnosis) | A self-limiting syndrome of 24–48 h apparently no sequelae. |
| Acute CNS depression Leukemia, aplastic anemia Dermatitis | Urinary phenol | Note that benzene, as with toluene and other solvents, can be monitored via its principal metabolite. |
| Acute CNS depression Chronic CNS problems such as memory loss | Urinary hippuric acid | |
| Irritation dermatitis | | |
| Irritation, pneumonitis, acute pulmonary edema (at high doses) Irritation Acute CNS depression | Methylhippuric acid in urine, xylene in expired air, xylene in blood | |
| Acute CNS depression MBK has been linked with peripheral neuropathy Dermatitis | Acetone in blood, urine, expired air (used as an index for exposure, not for diagnosis) | The ketone family demonstrates how a pattern of toxic responses (that is, CNS narcosis) may feature exceptions (i.e., MBK peripheral neuropathy). |

continued on next page

TABLE D-l: Continued

| Agent | Exposure | Route of Entry | Systems(s) Affected |
|---|---|---|---|
| Formaldehyde | Widely used as a germicide and a disinfectant in embalming and histopathology, for example, and in the manufacture of textiles, resins, and other products | Inhalation | Skin<br>Eye<br>Pulmonary |
| Trichloro-ethylene (TCE) | Solvent in metal degreasing, dry cleaning, food extraction; ingredient of paints, adhesives, varnishes, inks | Inhalation, percutaneous absorption | Nervous<br><br>Skin<br>Cardiovascular |
| Carbon tetrachloride | Solvent for oils, fats, lacquers, resins, varnishes, other materials; used as a degreasing and cleaning agent | Inhalation of vapor | Hepatic<br>Renal<br>CNS<br>Skin |
| Carbon disulfide | Solvent for lipids, sulfur, halogens, rubber, phosphorus, oils, waxes, and resins; manufacturing of organic chemicals, paints, fuels, explosives, viscose rayon | Inhalation of vapor, percutaneous absorption of liquid or vapor | Nervous<br><br>Renal<br><br>Cardiovascular<br><br>Skin<br>Reproductive |

| Primary Manifestations | Aids in Diagnosis[a] | Remarks |
|---|---|---|
| Irritant and contact dermatitis<br>Eye irritation<br>Respiratory tract irritation, asthma | Patch testing may be helpful for dermatitis | Recent animal tests have shown it to be a respiratory carcinogen. Confirmatory epidemiologic studies are in progress. |
| Acute CNS depression<br>Peripheral and cranial neuropathy<br>Irritation, dermatitis<br>Arrhythmias | Breath analysis for TCE | TCE is involved in an important pharmacological interaction. Within hours of ingesting alcoholic beverages, TCE workers experience flushing of the face, neck, shoulders, and back. Alcohol may also potentiate the CNS effects of TCE. The probable mechanism is competition for metabolic enzymes. |
| Toxic hepatitis<br>Oliguria or anuria<br>Acute CNS depression<br>Dermatitis | Expired air and blood levels | Carbon tetrachloride is the prototype for a wide variety of solvents that cause hepatic and renal damage. This solvent, like trichloroethylene, acts synergistically with ethanol. |
| Parkinsonism, psychosis, suicide<br>Peripheral neuropathies<br>Chronic nephritic and nephrotic syndromes<br>Acceleration or worsening of atherosclerosis; hypertension<br>Irritation; dermatitis<br>Menorrhagia and metrorrhagia | Iodine-azide reaction with urine (nonspecific since other bivalent sulfur compounds give a positive test); $CS_2$ in expired air, blood, and urine | A solvent with unusual multisystem effects, especially noted for its cardiovascular, renal, and nervous system actions. |

continued on next page

TABLE D-1: Continued

| Agent | Exposure | Route of Entry | Systems(s) Affected |
|-------|----------|----------------|---------------------|
| Stoddard solvent | Degreasing, paint thinning | Inhalation of vapor, percutaneous absorption of liquid | Skin<br><br>CNS |
| Ethylene glycol ethers (Ethylene glycol monoethyl ether— Cellosolve®) (Ethylene glycol monoethyl ether acetate—Cello- solve acetate) | The ethers are used as solvents for resins, paints, lacquers, varnishes, gum, perfume, dyes, and inks; the acetate derivatives are widely used as solvents and ingredients of lacquers, enamels, and adhesives. Exposure occurs in dry cleaning, plastic, ink, and lacquer manufacturing, and textile dying, among other processes. | Inhalation of vapor, percutaneous absorption of liquid | Reproductive, CNS, renal, liver |
| (Methyl- and butyl-substituted compounds such as ethylene glycol mono- methyl ether— Methyl Cellosolve®) | | | Hematopoietic CNS |
| Ethylene oxide | Used in the sterilization of medical equipment, in the fumigation of spices and other foodstuffs, and as a chemical intermediate | Inhalation | Skin<br>Eye<br><br>Respiratory tract<br>Nervous system |
| Dioxane | Used as a solvent for a variety of materials, including cellulose acetate, dyes, fats, greases, resins, polyvinyl polymers, varnishes, and waxes | Inhalation of vapor, percutaneous absorption of liquid | CNS<br><br><br>Renal<br>Liver |

| Primary Manifestations | Aids in Diagnosis[a] | Remarks |
|---|---|---|
| Dryness and scaling from defatting; dermatitis<br>Dizziness, coma, collapse (at high levels) | | A mixture of primarily aliphatic hydrocarbons, with some benzene derivatives and naphthenes. |
| | | Ethylene glycol ethers, as a class of chemicals, have been shown in animals to have adverse reproductive effects, including reduced sperm count and spontaneous abortion, as well as CNS, renal, and liver effects. |
| Pancytopenia<br>Fatigue, lethargy, nausea, headaches, anorexia, tremor, stupor (from encephalopathy) | | Effects primary associated with ethylene glycol monomethyl ether (Methyl Cellosolve®) |
| Dermatitis and frostbite<br>Severe irritation; possibly cataracts with prolonged exposure<br>Irritation<br>Peripheral neuropathy | | Recent animal tests have shown it to be carcinogenic and to cause reproductive abnormalities. Epidemiologic studies indicate that it may cause leukemia in exposed workers. |
| Drowsiness, dizziness, anorexia, headaches, nausea, vomiting, coma<br>Nephritis<br>Chemical hepatitis | | Dioxane has caused a variety of neoplasms in animals. |

continued on next page

TABLE D-1: Continued

| Agent | Exposure | Route of Entry | Systems(s) Affected |
|-------|----------|----------------|---------------------|
| Polychlorinated biphenyls (PCBs) | Formerly used as a di-electric fluid in electrical equipment and as a fire retardant coating on tiles and other products. New uses were banned in 1976, but much of the electrical equipment currently used still contains PCBs | Inhalation, ingestion, skin absorption | Skin Eye Liver |

**Irritant Gases**[c]

| Agent | Exposure | Route of Entry | Systems(s) Affected |
|-------|----------|----------------|---------------------|
| Ammonia | Refrigeration; petroleum refining; manufacturing of nitrogen-containing chemicals, synthetic fibers, dyes, and optics | Inhalation of gas | Upper respiratory tract |
| Hydrochloric acid | Chemical manufacturing; electroplating; tanning; metal pickling; petroleum extraction; rubber, photographic, and textile industries | Inhalation of gas or mist | Upper respiratory tract |
| Hydrofluoric acid | Chemical and plastic manufacturing; catalyst m petroleum refining; aqueous solution for frosting, etching, and polishing glass | Inhalation of gas or mist | Upper respiratory tract |
| Sulfur dioxide | Manufacturing of sulfur-containing chemicals; food and textile bleach; tanning; metal casting | Inhalation of gas, direct contact of gas or liquid phase on skin or mucosa | Middle respiratory tract |
| Chlorine | Paper and textile bleaching; water disinfection; chemical manufacturing; metal fluxing; detinning and dezincing iron | Inhalation of gas | Middle respiratory tract |

| Primary Manifestations | Aids in Diagnosis[a] | Remarks |
|---|---|---|
| Chloracne<br>Irritation<br>Toxic hepatitis | Serum PCB levels for chronic exposure | Animal studies have demonstrated that PCBs are carcinogenic. Epidemiologic studies of exposed workers are inconclusive. |
| Upper respiratory irritation | | Also irritant of eyes and moist skin. |
| Upper respiratory irritation | | Strong irritant of eyes, mucous membranes, and skin. |
| Upper respiratory irritation | | In solution, causes severe and painful burns of skin and can be fatal. |
| Bronchospasm (pulmonary edema or chemical pneumonitis in high dose) | Chest x ray, pulmonary function tests[d] | Strong irritant of eyes, mucous membranes, and skin. |
| Tracheobronchitis, pulmonary edema, pneumonitis | Chest x ray, pulmonary function tests | Chlorine combines with body moisture to form acids, which irritate tissues from nose to alveoli. |

continued on next page

TABLE D-1: Continued

| Agent | Exposure | Route of Entry | Systems(s) Affected |
|---|---|---|---|
| Ozone | Inert gas-shielded arc welding; food, water, and air purification; food and textile bleaching; emitted around high-voltage electrical equipment | Inhalation of gas | Lower respiratory tract |
| Nitrogen oxides | Manufacturing of acids, nitrogen-containing chemicals, explosives, and more; byproduct of many industrial processes | Inhalation of gas | Lower respiratory tract |
| Phosgene | Manufacturing and burning of isocyanates, and manufacturing of dyes and other organic chemicals; in metallurgy for ore separation; burning or heat source near trichloroethylene | Inhalation of gas | Lower respiratory tract |
| Isocyanates<br><br>TDI (toluene diisocyanate)<br><br>MDI (methylene diphenyldiiso-cyanate)<br><br>Hexamethylene diisocyanate and others | Polyuredhane manufacture; resin-binding systems in foundries; coating materials for wires; used certain types of paint | Inhalation of vapor | Predominantly lower respiratory tract |
| Asphyxiant gases<br>Simple asphyxiants: nitrogen hydrogen, methane, and others | Enclosed spaces in a variety of industrial settings | Inhalation of gas | CNS |

| Primary Manifestations | Aids in Diagnosis[a] | Remarks |
|---|---|---|
| Delayed pulmonary edema (generally 6-8 h following exposure) | Chest x ray, pulmonary function tests | Ozone has a free radical structure and can produce experimental chromosome aberrations; it may thus have carcinogenic potential. |
| Pulmonary irritation, bronchiolitis fibrosa obliterans ("silo filler's disease"), mixed obstructive-restrictive changes | Chest x ray, pulmonary function tests | |
| Delayed pulmonary edema (delay seldom longer than 12 h) | Chest x ray, pulmonary function tests | |
| Asthmatic reaction and accelerated loss of pulmonary function | Chest x ray, pulmonary function tests | Isocyanates are both respiratory tract "sensitizers" and irritants in the conventional sense. |
| Anoxia | $O_2$ in environment | No specific toxic effect; acts by displacing $O_2$. |

continued on next page

TABLE D-1: Continued

| Agent | Exposure | Route of Entry | Systems(s) Affected |
|---|---|---|---|
| **Chemical Asphyxiants** | | | |
| Carbon monoxide | Incomplete combustion in foundries, coke ovens, refineries, furnaces, and more | Inhalation of gas | Blood (hemoglobin) |
| Hydrogen sulfide | Used in manufacturing of sulfur-containing chemicals; produced in petroleum production; byproduct of petroleum product use; decay of organic matter | Inhalation of gas | CNS<br><br>Pulmonary |
| Cyanides | Metallurgy, electroplating | Inhalation of vapor, percutaneous absorption, ingestion | Cellular metabolic enzymes (especially cytochrome oxidase) |
| **Pesticides** | | | |
| Organo-phophates: malathion, parathion, and others | | Inhalation, ingestions, percutaneous absorption | Neuromuscular |
| Carbamates: carbaryl (Sevin) and others | | Inhalation, ingestion, percutaneous absorption | Neuromuscular |

| Primary Manifestations | Aids in Diagnosis[a] | Remarks |
|---|---|---|
| Headache; dizziness, double vision | Carboxy-hemoglobin | |
| Respiratory center paralysis, hypoventilation Respiratory tract irritation | $PaO_2$ | |
| Enzyme inhibition with metabolic asphyxia and death | $SCN^-$ in urine | |
| Cholinesterase inhibition, cholinergic symptoms: nausea and vomiting, salivation, diarrhea, headache, seating, meiosis, muscle fasciculations, seizures, unconsciousness, death | Refractoriness to atropine; plasma or red cell cholinesterase | As with many acute toxins, rapid treatment of organophosphate toxicity is imperative. Thus, diagnosis is often made based on history and a high index of suspicion rather than on biochemical tests. Treatment is atropine to block cholinergic effects and 2-PAM (2-pyridine-alsoxine meth-iodide) to reactivate cholinesterase. |
| Same as organophosphates | Plasma cholinesterase; urinary 1-naphthol (index of exposure) | Treatment of carbamate poisoning is the same as that of organo-phosphate poisoning except that 2-PAM is contraindicated. |

continued on next page

TABLE D-1: Continued

| Agent | Exposure | Route of Entry | Systems(s) Affected |
|---|---|---|---|
| Chlorinated hydrocarbons: chlordane, DDT, heptachlor, chlor-decone (Kepone), aldrin, dieldrin, uridine | | Ingestion, inhalation, percutaneous absorption | CNS |
| Bipyridyls: paraquat, diquat | | Inhalation, ingestion, percutaneous absorption | Pulmonary |

[a]Occupational and medical histories are in most instances, the most important aids in diagnosis.

[b]Zinc oxide is a prototype of agents that cause metal fume fever.

[c]The less water-soluble the gas, the deeper and more delayed its irritant effect.

| Primary Manifestations | Aids in Diagnosis[a] | Remarks |
|---|---|---|
| Stimulation or depression | Urinary organic chlorine, or *p*-chloro-phenol acetic acid | The chlorinated hydro-carbons may accumu-late in body lipid stores in large amounts. |
| Rapid massive fibrosis, only following paraquat ingestion | | An interesting toxin in that the major toxicity, pulmonary fibrosis, apparently occurs only after ingestion. |

[a]Pulmonary function tests are useful aids in diagnosis of irritant effects if the patient is subacutely or chronically ill.

SOURCE: Reprinted, with permission, from *Principles and Practice of Environmental Health*, A.B. Tarcher, ed. Copyright 1992 by Plenum Publishing Co.

TABLE D-2: Selected Work-Related Diseases, Disorders, and Conditions Associated with Various Agents, Industries, or Occupations: Infections, Malignant Neoplasms, and Hematological, Cardiovascular, Pulmonary, Neurological, and Miscellaneous Disorders

| Diseases, Disorders, and Conditions | Industry or Occupation | Agent |
|---|---|---|
| **Infections** | | |
| Anthrax | Shepherds, farmers, butchers, handlers of imported hides or fibers, veterinarians, veterinarian pathologists, weavers | *Bacillus anthraces* |
| Brucellosis | Farmers, shepherds, vets, lab and slaughterhouse workers | *Brucella abortus, suis* |
| Plague | Shepherds, farmers, ranchers, hunters, field geologists | *Yersinia pestis* |
| Hepatitis A | Day-care center, orphanage, and mental retardation institution staff, medical personnel | Hepatitis A virus |
| Hepatitis B | Nurses and aides, anesthesiologists, orphanage and mental institution staffs, medical lab workers, general dentists, oral surgeons, physicians | Hepatitis B virus |
| Hepatitis C (formerly included in non-A, non-B) | Same as hepatitis A and B | Hepatitis C virus |
| Ornithosis | Psittacine bird breeders, pet shop and zoo workers, poultry producers, vets | *Chlamydia psittaci* |
| Rabies | Veterinarians, game wardens, lab workers, farmers, ranchers, trappers | Rabies virus |
| Rubella | Medical personnel | Rubella virus |
| Tetanus | Farmers, ranchers | *Clostridium tetani* |
| Tuberculosis Pulmonary | Physicians, medical personnel, medical lab workers | *Mycobacterium tuberculosis* |
| Tuberculosis Silicotuberculosis | Quarrymen, sandblasters, silica processors, miners, foundry workers, ceramic industry | Silicon dioxide (silica), *M. tuberculosis* |

## TABLE D-2: Continued

| Diseases, Disorders, and Conditions | Industry or Occupation | Agent |
|---|---|---|
| Tularemia | Hunters, fur handlers, sheep industry, cooks, veterinarians, ranchers, veterinarian pathologists | *Francisella tularensis* |

**Malignant Neoplasms**

| | | |
|---|---|---|
| Bladder | Rubber and dye workers | Benzidine, 1- and 2-naphthyl-amine, auramine, magenta, 4-aminobiphenyl, 4-nitrophenyl |
| Bone | Dial painters, radium chemists and processors | Radium |
| Kidney and other urinary organs | Coke oven workers | Coke oven emissions |
| Liver | Vinyl chloride polymerization industry | Vinyl chloride monomer |
| Liver hemangiosarcoma | Vintners | Arsenical pesticides |
| Lung, bronchial, tracheal | Asbestos industry, users | Asbestos |
| | Topside coke oven workers | Coke oven emissions |
| | Uranium and fluorspar miners | Radon daughters |
| | Chromium producers, processors, users | Chromates |
| | Smelters | Arsenic |
| | Mustard gas formulators | Mustard gas |
| | Ion-exchange resin makers, chemists | Bis(chloro-methyl)-ether, chloromethyl methyl ether |
| Nasal cavity | Woodworkers, furniture makers | Hardwood dusts |
| | Boot and shoe industry | Unknown |
| | Radium chemists and processors, dial painters | Radium |
| | Chromium producers, processors, users | Chromates |
| | Nickel smelting and refining | Nickel Asbestos |

continued on next page

## TABLE D-2: Continued

| Diseases, Disorders, and Conditions | Industry or Occupation | Agent |
|---|---|---|
| Peritoneal, pleural mesothelioma | Asbestos industry, users | Asbestos |
| Scrotal | Automatic lathe operators, metalworkers | Mineral, cutting oils |
|  | Coke oven workers, petroleum refiners, tar distillers | Soots and tars, tar distillates |
| **Hematological Disorders** | | |
| Agranulocytosis or neutropenia | Workers exposed to benzene | Benzene |
|  | Explosives, pesticide industries | Phosphorus |
|  | Pesticide, pigment, pharmaceutical industries | Inorganic arsenic |
| Anemia Aplastic | Explosives manufacturing | TNT |
|  | Workers exposed to benzene | Benzene |
|  | Radiologists, radium chemists, dial painters | Ionizing radiation |
| Anemia Hemolytic, nonautoimmune | Whitewashing and leather industry | Copper sulfate |
|  | Electrolytic processes, arsenical ore smelting | Arsine |
|  | Plastics industry | Trimellitic anhydride |
|  | Dye, celluloid, resin industries | Naphthalene |
| Leukemia Acute lymphoid | Rubber industry | Unknown |
|  | Radiologists | Ionizing radiation |
| Leukemia Acute myeloid | Workers exposed to benzene | Benzene |
|  | Radiologists | Ionizing radiation |
| Leukemia Erythroleukemia | Workers exposed to benzene | Benzene |
| Methemoglobinemia | Explosives, dye industries | Aromatic amino and nitro compounds (e.g., aniline, TNT, nitroglycerin) |

## TABLE D-2: Continued

| Diseases, Disorders, and Conditions | Industry or Occupation | Agent |
| --- | --- | --- |

### Cardiovascular Disorders

| | | |
| --- | --- | --- |
| Angina | Auto mechanics, foundry workers, wood finishers, traffic control, driving in heavy traffic | Carbon monoxide |
| Arrhythmias | Metal cleaning, solvent use, refrigerator maintenance | Solvents, fluorocarbons |
| Raynaud's phenomenon | Lumberjacks, chain sawyers, grinders, chippers | Whole-body or segmental vibration |
| (secondary) | Vinyl chloride polymerization | Vinyl chloride monomer |

### Pulmonary Disorders

| | | |
| --- | --- | --- |
| Alveolitis (extrinsic, allergic) | Farmer's lung bagassosis, bird-breeder's lung,suberosis, maltworker's lung, mushroom worker's lung, maple bark disease, cheese-washer's lung, coffee-worker's lung, fish-meal-worker's lung, furrier's lung, sequoiosis, woodworker's lung, miller's lung | Various agents |
| Asbestosis | Asbestos workers, users | Asbestos |
| Asthma (extrinsic) | Jewelry, alloy, catalyst makers | Platinum |
| | Polyurethane, adhesive, paint workers | Isocyanates |
| | Alloy, catalyst, refinery workers | Chromium, cobalt |
| | Solderers | Aluminum soldering flux |
| | Plastic, dye, insecticide makers | Phthalic anhydride |
| | Foam workers, latex makers, biologists | Formaldehyde |
| | Printing industry | Gum arabic |
| | Nickel platers | Nickel sulfate |
| | Bakers | Flour |
| | Plastics industry | Trimellitic anhydride |
| | Woodworkers, furniture makers | Red cedar, wood dusts |
| | Detergent formulators | Bacillus-derived exoenzymes |
| | Animal handlers | Animal dander |

continued on next page

## TABLE D-2: Continued

| Diseases, Disorders, and Conditions | Industry or Occupation | Agent |
|---|---|---|
| Beryllium disease (chronic) | Beryllium alloy, ceramic, cathode-ray tube, nuclear reactor workers | Beryllium |
| Bronchitis, pneumonitis, pulmonary edema (acute) | Refrigeration, fertilizer, oil-refining industries | Ammonia |
| | Alkali, beach industries | Chlorine |
| | Silo fillers, arc welders, nitric acid workers | Nitrogen oxides |
| | Paper, refrigeration, oil-refining industries | Sulfur dioxide |
| | Cadmium smelters, processors | Cadmium |
| | Plastics industry | Trimellitic anhydride |
| Byssinosis | Cotton industry | Cotton, flax, hemp, cotton-synthetic dusts |
| Pneumoconiosis | Coal miners, bauxite workers | Coal dust, bauxite fumes |
| Silicosis | Mining, metal, and ceramic industries, quarrymen, sand blasters, silica processors | Silica |
| Talcosis | Talc processors | Talc |

**Neurological Disorders**

| | | |
|---|---|---|
| Cerebellar ataxia | Chemical industry | Toluene |
| | Electrolytic chlorine production, battery manufacturing, fungicide formulators | Organic mercury |
| Encephalitis (toxic) | Battery, smelter, foundry workers | Lead |
| | Electrolytic chlorine production, battery manufacturing, fungicide formulators | Organic, inorganic mercury |
| Neuropathy (toxic and inflammatory) | Pesticide, pigment, pharmaceutical industries | Arsenic, arsenic compounds |
| | Furniture refinishers, degreasers | Hexane |
| | Plastic-coated-fabric workers | Methyl butyl ketone |
| | Explosives industry | TNT |
| | Rayon manufacturing | Carbon disulfide |
| | Plastics, hydraulics, coke industries | Tri-o-cresyl phosphate |

## TABLE D-2: Continued

| Diseases, Disorders, and Conditions | Industry or Occupation | Agent |
|---|---|---|
| Neuropathy (toxic and inflammatory) | Battery, smelter, foundry workers | Inorganic lead |
| | Dentists, chloralkali workers | Inorganic mercury |
| | Chloralkali, fungicide, battery workers | Organic mercury |
| | Plastics, paper manufacture | Acrylamide |
| Parkinson's disease (secondary) | Manganese processors, battery manufacturing, welders | Manganese |
| | Internal combustion engine industries | Carbon monoxide |

**Miscellaneous**

| | | |
|---|---|---|
| Abdominal pain | Battery manufacturing, enamelers, smelter, painters, ceramics workers, plumbers, welders | Lead |
| Cataract | Microwave, radar technicians | Microwaves |
| | Explosives industry | TNT |
| | Radiologists | Ionizing radiation |
| | Blacksmiths, glass blowers, bakers | Infrared radiation |
| | Moth repellent formulators, fumigators | Naphthalene |
| | Explosives, dye, herbicide, pesticide industries | Dinitrophenol, dinitro-o-cresol |
| Dermatitis (contact, allergic) | Adhesives, sealants, and plastics industries, leather tanning, poultry dressing, fish packing, boat building and repair, electroplating, metal cleaning, machining, housekeeping | Irritants (cutting oils, solvents, phenol, acids, alkalies, detergents, fibrous glass), allergens (nickel, epoxy resins, chromates, formaldehyde, dyes, rubber products) |
| Headache | Firefighters, foundry workers, wood finishers, dry cleaners, traffic control, driving in heavy traffic | Carbon monoxide, solvents |
| Hepatitis (toxic) | Solvent users, dry cleaners, plastics industry | Carbon tetrachloride, chloroform, tetrachloroethane trichloroethylene |

continued on next page

TABLE D-2: Continued

| Diseases, Disorders, and Conditions | Industry or Occupation | Agent |
| --- | --- | --- |
| Hepatitis (toxic) | Explosives and dye industries | Phosphorus, TNT |
| | Fire and waterproofing additive formulators | Chloronaphthalene |
| | Plastics formulators | 4,4-Methylene-dianiline |
| | Fumigators, gasoline and fire-extinguisher formulators | Ethylene dibromide |
| | Disinfectant, fumigant, synthetic resin formulators | Cresol |
| Inner ear damage | Various | Excessive noise |
| Infertility (male) | Formulators | Kepone |
| | Producers, formulators, applicators | 1,2-Dibromo-3-chloropropane |
| Psychosis (acute) | Gasoline, seed, and fungicide workers, wood preservation, rayon manufacturing | Lead (especially organic), mercury, carbon disulfide |
| Renal failure (acute, chronic) | Battery manufacturing, plumbers, solderers | Inorganic lead |
| | Electrolytic processes, arsenical ore smelting | Arsine |
| | Battery manufacturing, jewelers, dentists | Inorganic mercury |
| | Fluorocarbon, fire-extinguisher formulators | Carbon tetrachloride |
| | Antifreeze manufacturing | Ethylene glycol |

SOURCE: Reprinted, with permission, from *Principles and Practice of Environmental Medicine*, Tarcher, AB, ed. Copyright 1992 by Plenum Publishing Co.

## TABLE D-3: Selected Job Categories, Exposures, and Associated Work-Related Diseases and Conditions

| Job Categories | Exposures | Work-Related Diseases and Conditions |
|---|---|---|
| Agricultural workers | Pesticides, infectious agents, gases, sunlight | Pesticide poisoning, "farmer's lung," skin cancer |
| Anesthetists | Anesthetic gases | Reproductive effects, cancer |
| Animal handlers | Infectious agents, allergens | Asthma |
| Automobile workers | Asbestos, plastics, lead, solvents | Asbestosis, dermatitis |
| Bakers | Flour | Asthma |
| Battery makers | Lead, arsenic | Lead poisoning, cancer |
| Butchers | Vinyl plastic fumes | "Meat wrappers' asthma" |
| Caisson workers | Pressurized work environments | "Caisson disease," "the bends" |
| Carpenters | Wood dust, wood preservatives, adhesives | Nasopharyngeal cancer, dermatitis |
| Cement workers | Cement dust, metals | Dermatitis, bronchitis |
| Ceramic workers | Talc, clays | Pneumoconiosis |
| Demolition workers | Asbestos, wood dust | Asbestosis |
| Drug manufacturers | Hormones, nitroglycerin, etc. | Reproductive effects |
| Dry cleaners | Solvents | Liver disease, dermatitis |
| Dye workers | Dyestuffs, metals, solvents | Bladder cancer, dermatitis |
| Embalmers | Formaldehyde, infectious agents | Dermatitis |
| Felt makers | Mercury, polycyclic hydrocarbons | Mercuralism |
| Foundry workers | Silica, molten metals | Silicosis |
| Glass workers | Heat, solvents, metal powders | Cataracts |
| Hospital workers | Infectious agents, cleansers, radiation | Infections, accidents |
| Insulators | Asbestos, fibrous glass | Asbestosis, lung cancer, mesothelioma |

## TABLE D-3: Continued

| Job Categories | Exposures | Work-Related Diseases and Conditions |
|---|---|---|
| Jack hammer operators | Vibration | Raynaud phenomenon |
| Lathe operators | Metal dusts, cutting oils | Lung disease, cancer |
| Laundry workers | Bleaches, soaps, alkalies | Dermatitis |
| Lead burners | Lead | Lead poisoning |
| Miners (coal, hard rock, metals, etc.) | Talc, radiation, metals, coal dust, silica | Pneumoconiosis, lung cancer |
| Natural gas workers | Polycyclic hydrocarbons | Lung cancer |
| Nuclear workers | Radiation, plutonium | Metal poisoning, cancer |
| Office workers | Poor lighting, poorly designed equipment | Joint problems, eye problems |
| Painters | Paints, solvents, spackling compounds | Neurologic problems |
| Paper makers | Acids, alkalies, solvents, metals | Lung disorders, dermatitis |
| Petroleum workers | Polycyclic hydrocarbons, catalysts, zeolites | Cancer, pneumoconiosis |
| Plumbers | Lead, solvents, asbestos | Lead poisoning |
| Railroad workers | Creosote, sunlight, oils, solvents | Cancer, dermatitis |
| Seamen | Sunlight, asbestos | Cancer, accidents |
| Smelter workers | Metals, heat, sulfur dioxide, arsenic | Cancer |
| Steel workers | Heat, metals, silica | Cataracts, heat stroke |
| Stone cutters | Silica | Silicosis |
| Textile workers | Cotton dust, fabrics, finishers, dyes, carbon disulfide | Byssinosis, dermatitis, psychosis |
| Varnish makers | Solvents, waxes | Dermatitis |
| Vineyard workers | Arsenic, pesticides | Cancer, dermatitis |
| Welders | Fumes, nonionizing radiation | Lead poisoning, cataracts |

SOURCE: Reprinted, with permission, from *Principles and Practice of Environmental Medicine*, A.B. Tarcher, ed. Copyright 1992 by Plenum Publishing Co.

# E

# Focus Group Summary and List of Participants

The following is a compilation of responses from focus groups that were convened by individual members of the IOM Committee on Enhancing Environmental Health in Nursing Practice. Twelve (12) focus groups were held with nurses in California, Iowa, Massachusetts, New Jersey, North Carolina, South Carolina, Texas, Washington, DC, and Louisiana.

Participants included specialists in the fields of occupational health, nurse practitioner and public health nursing faculty, practicing public health nurses, practicing family nurse practitioners, nursing doctoral students, nurses representing the American Organization of Nurse Executives, and representatives from the American Association of Colleges of Nursing.

**1. What comes to mind with the words "environmental health (EH) issues"?**
Responses to this question fell into eight major categories.

*Nursing Practice Issues*
- Absence of EH in current scope of nursing practice, including primary care.
- Issue of "jurisdiction" was commonly mentioned. Nursing not linked with public sector in addressing EH issues.
- Reimbursement for EH services (how, by whom?)

- Recall early PHN practice, where health problems were related to poor sanitation
- Detection, assessment, evaluation, treatment of hazardous substances' toxic effects
- Accident prevention and elimination of hazards
- Pollutants from health care industry
- Practicing with the unit of analysis being the community rather than the individual

*Psycho-social Issues*
- Inner city violence and poverty at epidemic levels (**mentioned by almost all)
- Hostile, life threatening environments created by crime
- Psychological effects of overcrowding, high density living (condos)
- Cultural issues around food and water contamination
- Environmental racism (burden of environmental hazards greatest on poor and minorities)
- Violence—family, community and workplace

*Public Awareness*
- Heightened public awareness about environmental hazards
- Teaching kids to recycle, but not health effects
- Media interest, expense

*Legal and Ethical Concerns*
- Conflicts between business and well-being of community
- EH legislation without funding to enforce
- Control and dissemination of information
- Conflict in consumer values—want technology, but not risks
- Cost of intervention vs. prevention
- Rights of the individual—to live in environment of choice, NRA and gun control
- Refer and forget—lack of accountability and continuity in addressing these issues

*Scientific/Research Issues*
- Cause and effect not often clear.
- Problems identifying causative agent(s) for illnesses that appear environmentally related.
- What is burden (or degree) of human illness/dysfunction that is associated with environmental conditions?
- Interaction of various conditions that result in illness

- Mechanism of environmental hazards in causing or contributing to disease
- Hazard control mechanisms inadequate
- Emphasis is more (too much?) on toxicology than society and community environs.

*Concern About Specific Environments*
- Hospitals and indoor air pollution
- Housing, homelessness
- Contamination of community by local industry
- Urban problems—violence, stress, crowding
- Rural health—lack capacity for assessments and referrals (lack of money)
- Definition of environment needs to include concepts of economics and power

*Concern About Specific Hazards*
**Sanitation**
Air, water and waste management were primary concerns overall

- Water and air pollution (indoor and outdoor) most frequently cited issues
- Sanitation in general
- Contamination of soil and play areas
- Contamination of seafood and recreational waters
- Contamination of drinking and recreational water by irrigation, farm chemical, and urban runoff

**Other Hazards**
- All types: chemical, biological, physical, mechanical, psycho-social
- Waste management and toxic waste (mentioned by more than half of groups)
- Fleas, mosquitoes, and pesticides
- Lead-based paint
- Sick buildings
- Farm safety
- Electromagnetic fields
- Noise (mentioned by more than half of the groups)
- Ozone depletion and UV-B exposure
- Natural disasters (tornadoes, fires, etc.)
- Workplace technology creating hazards to health
- Ergonomics

- Deforestation
- Foodborne disease
- Strip mining and contamination of wells
- Radiation exposures
- Disease vectors and pest management

*Specific Health Conditions*
- TB
- Gulf War syndrome
- Sick building syndrome
- Legionnaires disease; childhood asthma; increasing incidence of allergic reactions
- Carpal tunnel syndrome

## 2.   *How* are nurses involved with EH?

*Education* (most frequently cited role)
- Accessing and disseminating info. regarding EH factors in health and illness
- Prevention oriented ed. on individual, worker, family and community basis
- Keeping track of local resources and distributing this info (as go between)
- Relaying standards and regulations to employers/employees
- Hygiene, immunization, risks, injury control, pica appetite
- Educate other team members/disciplines who are more narrowly focused

*Advocacy*
- Work with community, environmental groups, local government
- Legislative lobbying
- Reporting community hazards
- Ideally, all nurses should be advocates for safer environments
- Involved in implementing policy

*How/Where Involvement Occurs*
- Via referrals from public sector
- Joint inspection of home, community, workplace
- ER, OH, and CH practice centers
- Involved in regulating teams
- Nurse is first to get complaint, then becomes involved in case management

*In Routine Practice and Research*
- First line problem identification; taking O/E histories
- Identify link between illness and environmental condition
- Recording and designing interventions, evaluation of outcomes
- Implementing medical screening exams (e.g., childhood lead, worker exposures such as pesticides, solvents, pharmaceuticals). Individual and population based.
- Demonstrate links between cost effectiveness and reducing hazards at work
- Work as interdisciplinary team member (***many groups commented on this)
- Focus on prevention, advocacy and as knowledgeable resource
- Research in environmental science and technology
- Suggest avenues of recourse, make recommendations to improve work conditions

*Environmental Assessment*
Although this is "routine practice" for some, it was mentioned so frequently and in such varied contexts, I made it a separate sub-section.

- Assessment of patients' environment, via history taking and on-site
- Identify exposures
- Field assessments as component of other ongoing intervention
- Extension of role into community and worker's family situation to identify problems related to community, home and workplace exposures

*Other*
- Nurses are not involved if not OHN, PHN or CHN
- Hospitals are poorest model of workplace safety/control of hazards. Hazardous but notviewed as such. Many "unempowered nurses," especially in hospital setting.
- If EH issues raised at work (hospitals included), often get squelched by administration.
- Nurses familiar with holistic approach, have advantage of interacting on personal level.


## 3. Other ways nurses could be involved?

- Generating data systems for environmental assessment and outcomes

- Designing "critical paths" which include environmental assessment
- Impact studies (consumer goods, land use)
- Increase visibility of issues via PSAs, working with community groups
- Work with professional associations
- Push for inclusion in interdisciplinary discussions
- More general education of public; publish in lay publications
- More thorough home assessments
- Become more involved with community, EH groups, corporate education
- More collaboration within nursing, share information with each other, e.g., PHN could work with ER nurse on issues like violence
- Move CH education to early part of nursing ed. so there is less separation between hospital and CH practice
- Educate, but also move political system. Law changes behavior more effectively than public education, e.g., bike helmet and seat belt laws.
- Revolutionize nursing ed. to focus more on social justice and critical thinking
- Serve as role models, and develop role expectations such that attention to EH is routine

**4. What would be gained with increased involvement and attention to EH issues?**

- Big change in HC delivery system, perspectives of medicine and community
- Role of nurse would change, they would have some architectural input in HC system.
    Amplifier effect would occur: 1) make smarter consumer, voter, taxpayer and thus 2) shape behavior of industry and business.
- Nurses and clients will be better able to think at a system level to effect change
- Primary prevention would be enhanced
- Decrease health care costs over long term, with earlier detection of "real" problem or etiology of disease, and interventions that address causative factors as well as medical symptoms.
- More holistic approach
- Nurses would become resource brokers
- Increasing power of lay-groups, if nurses openly stand with them and educate them.

- Consumer would be more prevention oriented
- Nurses would become a political voice for disenfranchised, at-risk peoples
- Increase scientific knowledge base about environmental exposure and disease
- More funding for EH practice, education and research — as knowledge base builds

### 5.  Drawbacks to enhancing EH in nursing practice?

- *Will be difficult to change practice and education:*

    -    Nurses don't know "what they don't know," thus cannot understand impacts of enhancing knowledge base about EH issues
    -    Nursing curricula already full
    -    No faculty expertise in this area, and curricula is driven (in part) by this
    -    Practicing nurses already spread too thin, no time to add new routine duties
    -    Will require "revolution" or "new paradigm" of nursing education and practice based on systems level approach and/or critical thinking
    -    May require redrawing the picture of nursing ed., rather than just adding content
    -    No reimbursement structure for these activities
    -    Be careful about creating expectations of quick fixes and easy solutions to EH problems.

- *Social and Economic Issues*

    -    Employers and employment may be threatened by nurses speaking out, drawing attention to issues
    -    Turf battles rather than interdisciplinary collaboration may result.
    -    Crusader image, can be portrayed negatively by peers, administrators, media
    -    Backlash from political orientation: stereotyping and further division among nurses

### 6. What must be done to include EH in nursing practice?

*Nursing Education Issues*
- Revamp nursing education: either add on EH piece, integrate it into other components, or include part of total revision of nursing curricula
- Develop faculty expertise
- Create new specialty in EH at graduate level (?)
- "Market" or educate nursing faculty and administrators about magnitude of EH problems, and value of creating more knowledgeable nursing workforce in this area
- Provide EH education at all levels of nursing education, and CE for current workforce.
- CE must be ongoing as environmental health knowledge base expands
- Begin to introduce earth science terms in (or in preparation for) nursing curricula
- Two or three nursing schools need to take the lead, pilot revision of curricula

*Nursing Practice/Professional Approaches*
- Educate administrators, CEOs, corporate officials about role nurses can take in resolution of EH problems
- Demonstrate cost-benefit of interventions (e.g. primary prevention), to administrators, government officials, and legislators
- Develop reimbursement structure for nursing EH interventions, e.g., working with insurance industry, change in NANDA codes
- Amend ANA definition of nursing, NLN accrediting criteria
- Amend credentialing/licensure exams to include EH content
- Amend some specialty practice area definitions, e.g., CHN, PHN
- Build coalitions with other disciplines for education and practice of EH

*National Legislative Initiatives/Federal Government Role*
- Create national info. systems with data elements that trigger indepth examination of environmental exposures (e.g., for asthma, lead poisoning, birth defects)
- Develop funding mechanism to support nursing expertise/faculty development in EH
- Shift health care funding priorities toward preventive, public health interventions

### 7. Barriers to enhancing EH in nursing practice?

* Lack of time in routine practice situations
* Lack of faculty expertise to teach content
* Lack of administrative commitment to and knowledge about EH issues
* Absence of EH content in credentialing, licensure, and accrediting systems
* Lack of reimbursement structure
* Nurses may have difficulty in employing non-traditional interventions. Want to know, why learn about something (EH issues) if there are no clear solutions, or clearly defined and proven nursing interventions to resolve problems.
* Nursing job and role descriptions are often narrow, with discreet description of duties
* Lack of funding to build nursing faculty and existing workforce expertise
* Nurses are barriers; "buying in" to EH as important to practice; need to see how knowledge will benefit them, help them do their job
* Consequences of speaking out (social and economic)

### 8. How to overcome barriers?

*Educate current workforce*

Alter basic nursing curricula
* Identify common threads and basics
* Examine models of practice that are successful
* Mandate competencies in accreditation of ed. programs
* Include environmental risk in nursing assessment
* Need some schools of nursing to test a new paradigm
* Create new specialists and expertise

*Educate nursing deans, faculty, preceptors*

*Funding and resource development*
* Make funding of health professionals a mandatory component of other federal funding related to EH
* Federal and foundation funding
* Work with national professional organizations to create initiatives in EH education

*Develop scientific basis of EH practice*
- Identify, characterize and control of EH hazards
- Initiate national data collection systems to 1) Further document scope of problem, 2) Identify populations at risk and develop and evaluate interventions, 3) Provide quantifiable justification for funding (nursing) research and education in EH

*Socialization of Nurses*
- Advocate EH for nurses on the job, before they even enter practice
- Develop multidisciplinary programs, projects to address EH.

*Collaborate*
- Empower nurses; impart knowledge and techniques for empowering community groups, workers, parents, etc.

*Gain support from those with power to change funding, legislation, workplace policy*
- Educate govt. officials, consumers re. need for changes
- Take more business oriented approach to EH; define what customer wants
- Consciousness raising: family and peers, as well as public

### 9. Who needs to be involved?

(From most to least frequently cited)
- Deans, faculty and schools of nursing and public health
- Health care providers (nurses, MDs, related disciplines)
- Policy makers, legislators, public officials
- Industry, employers, CEOs
- Nursing administrators
- National nursing organizations, State Boards of Nursing, Accrediting Bodies
- Federal sector, private foundations, insurers
- Consumers, community activists, environmental groups (even extremists, because nurses mediate well, good brokers and coalition builders)

### 10. What educational methods appropriate for this content?

*Traditional Methods*
- Classroom; integrate in health assessment courses; literature—update textbooks to include EH; merge PH with nursing content

*Critical Thinking/Problem Solving*
- Case Study
- Systems paradigm that focuses on decision making
- Specific Content on Environmental Risk

*Site visits*
Internships, precepting, role models, interdisciplinary, community groups

*Multi-media*
Telecommunication, interactive video, visual aids, newsletters, media (with subliminal messages?), the arts

*Workshops/Seminars*
- Visiting workshops, professional conference topic, faculty education programs, lunch time seminars, CE, informal (fun) ways.
- Make efforts specialized to cultural concerns and relevance to client
- New view of world; view people in their context

**11. At what level(s) of nursing education should EH content be included?**

(Number in parenthesis indicates number of times cited by focus groups)
- All basic nursing education—core component (8)
- CE and Post-graduate (4)
- Specialization at graduate level (3)
- Baccalaureate and Masters (AD has no room) (1)
- All specialties (1)
- At ADN level teach assessment only (1)
- CEOHN certification (1)
- Sophisticated systems thinking and pop. based assessment may not be possible at basic baccalaureate level; perhaps nursing ed paradigm changes need to be made

**12. Which nursing specialties might be involved in EH research?**

(Number in parenthesis indicates number of times specialty was mentioned)

- PHN and CHN (7)
- All nurses, all specialties (5)
- Occupational Health Nurses (5)
- Maternal and Child Health (4)
- Primary Care (3)
- Pediatrics
- Oncology (2)
- ER (2)
- Mental Health/Psych (2)
- School Nurses, Nurse Educators, Geriatrics, Home Health, Cruise
Ship Nurses, Employee Health, Insurance Industry Nurses, Genetics (1)

## FOCUS GROUP PARTICIPANTS

Gale B. Adcock, M.S.N., F.N.P., C.S.
SAS Institute Inc.

Carole A. Anderson, Ph.D.

Ohio State University

Rhonda Anderson, M.P.A., R.N.,
    F.A.A.N.
Hartford Hospital

Mary Aquilino, Ph.D., R.N., F.N.P.
University of Iowa

Judith Baigis-Smith, R.N., Ph.D.,
    B.S.N.
Georgetown University

B.J. Bartleson, M.S., R.N.
University of California, Davis

Timothy J. Bevelacqua, M.N.,
    R.N., C.N.A.
St. Luke's Episcopal Hospital

Marjorie Beyers, Ph.D., R.N.,
    F.A.A.N.
American Organization of Nurse
    Executives

Christine Bolla, M.S., Ph.D.
    (candidate)
University of California, San
    Francisco

Pam Bromley, M.S.M., R.N.
Saint Alphonsus Regional Medical
    Center

Karen A. Brykczynski, R.N., C.S.,
    F.N.P., D.N.Sc.
University of Texas

Kathleen Clark, Ph.D., R.N., F.N.P
University of Iowa

Pat Clinton, M.A., R.N., P.N.P.
University of Iowa

Joan Duran, B.A., M.A., B.S.N,
Contra Costa County, CA

M. Louise Fitzpatrick, Ed.D.
Villanova University

Patty Franklin, C.P.N.P.
National Association of Pediatric
    Nurse Associates and
    Practitioners

Grace Gainey, R.N.
Kershaw County, S.C.

Kristine Gebbie, R.N., Dr.P.H.
Columbia University School of
    Nursing

Barbara Goldrick, R.N., Ph.D.
Georgetown University

Lisa Haley, R.N., B.S.N., C.O.H.N.
AT&T

Sue Hudec, M.S.N., R.N.
Veterans Affairs Medical Center

Phoebe Joseph, R.N., B.S.N.
Georgetown University Hospital

Alice Kamin, R.N.
Sumter County, S.C.

Carole Kelly, M.S., Ph.D.
    (candidate)
University of California, San
    Francisco

Nancy J. Krombach, R.N. M.S.N.,
    F.N.P., C.S.
SAS Institute Inc.

Jane Leonard, R.N.C., M.S.N.
University of Texas

Andrea R. Lindell, D.N.Sc.
University of Cincinnati

Sally Lusk, Ph.D., M.P.H., F.A.A.N
Association of Community Health
    Nursing
    Educators

Wendy J. Malone, B.S.N., P.H.N.
Contra Costa County, CA

Ann Marie McCarthy, Ph.D., R.N.,
    P.N.P.
University of Iowa

Judith McFarlane, Dr.P.H.,
    F.A.A.N.
American Nurses Association

Robert Mehl, B.S.N., R.N., C.S.N.
National Association of School
    Health Nurses

Ellen S. Meyer, B.S., R.N.,
    C.O.H.N.
Digital Equipment Corporation

Virginia M. Minnicello, M.S., R.N.,
    C.O.H.N.
Beth Israel Hospital

Marian Moody, R.N.
Clarendon County, S.C.

Wendy Myler, R.N., B.S.,
    C.O.H.N., C.C.M
Digital Equipment Corporation

Martha Nelson, M.S., Ph.D.
    (candidate)
University of California, San
    Francisco

Mary Ann Nugent, R.N.
Wateree Health District, S.C.

Aroha Page, M.S.N., Ph.D.
    (candidate)
University of California, San
    Francisco

Maureen Paul, M.D., M.P.H.
American College of Occupational
    and Environmental Medicine

Kathy Ras, R.N.
AT&T

Libby Rembert, R.N.
Lee County, S.C.

Carole Scott, R.N.
Sumter County, S.C.

Willie Swanson, B.A., B.S.N.
Contra Costa County, CA

Gale N. Touger, R.N., F.N.P., C.S.
SAS Institute Inc.

Patricia Travers, M.S., R.N.,
    C.O.H.N.
Digital Equipment Corporation

Karen Van Varick-McGuire, R.N.,
    B.S.N., C.O.H.N.
Johnson and Johnson

Mary Lou Wassell, M.Ed., R.N.,
    C.O.H.N.
American Association of
    Occupational Health Nurses

Barbareta A. Welch, M.S.N., R.N.,
    F.N.P., C.S.
SAS Institute Inc.

Joan A. West, M.A., P.H.N.
Contra Costa County, CA

Dot Williams, R.N.
Sumter County, S.C.

# F

# Nursing Advocacy at the Policy Level: Strategies and Resources[*]

Dealing with the environmental aspects of health is very likely to lead nurses into some form of *policy advocacy*. For example, nurses who encounter multiple cases of childhood lead poisoning in a particular neighborhood might see a need to develop community-based programs for lead screening, health education, and hazard abatement. In communities affected by toxic waste, nurses might be asked by residents to take sides publicly in partisan debates, answer reporters' questions, and perhaps give expert testimony in court cases. Nurses concerned that their patients' asthma is being worsened by industrial air pollution might decide to lobby for stronger regulation and enforcement of existing air quality standards, or to give technical support to citizens' groups protesting the pollution.

This kind of advocacy, aimed at influencing social institutions rather than securing services for individuals, represents uncharted territory for most nurses. Even those with a strong interest in policy advocacy may lack the information and experience needed to proceed with confidence. Accordingly, in the Institute of Medicine's report on *Nursing, Health and the Environment*, we have included this Appendix section as a support for nurses who wish to know more about concepts, strategies, and resources related to advocacy at the policy level.

---

[*]Appendix F, *Nursing Advocacy at the Policy Level: Strategies and Resources*, was written by Carolyn Needleman, an IOM committee member, for this report. Dr. Needleman is a Professor at the Graduate School of Social Work and Social Research at Bryn Mawr College.

## LEVELS OF ADVOCACY: CASE AND CLASS

In thinking about what advocacy means in the context of nursing practice, a clear distinction needs to be made between "*case advocacy*" directed at individual patients, and "*class advocacy*" directed at changing policies and social conditions.

Case advocacy is well known to nursing professionals, being part of the field's traditions and continuing professional values (Cary, 1992; Gadow and Schroeder, 1995; Nelson, 1988; Kohnke, 1982; Winslow, 1984; Marks, 1985). Nurses are accustomed to advocating for individual patients and families to secure needed services and solve problems related to the particular case. Over the years the concept of case advocacy has undergone an important evolution in nursing practice, gradually coming to include more emphasis on client empowerment. Shifting from its early meaning of *interceding* on behalf of those who could not or would not help themselves, advocacy for patients has now come to involve a more complex set of activities placing the nurse in *mediator* and *promoter* roles (Cary, 1992). These contemporary case advocacy roles emphasize client self-determination. They put a premium on *informing* and *supporting* clients, enabling them to define and act in terms of their own best interests (Kohnke, 1982). While in principle the "client" can be a community as well as an individual, the skills and objectives of case advocacy tend to stress better coping strategies, negotiation, and increasing access to existing resources in order to get health problems solved in the absence of major system change.

Class advocacy, a more overtly political approach, is quite different. Instead of focusing mainly on the client's opportunity choices, class advocacy focuses on changing the system of opportunities itself to further the interests of larger groups, organizations, or communities. The advocate acts as a catalyst to alter existing policies, institutional systems, laws, or patterns of resource allocation in ways that potentially benefit many individuals. This kind of advocacy can be done in ways that challenge the system *directly*, or it can be done *indirectly* behind the scenes (see Needleman and Needleman, 1974).

The following example, borrowed in part from Cary (1992), is a good illustration of how both case advocacy and class advocacy might be used by nurses faced with an environmental health problem:

> A community health nurse doing immunizations at a homeless shelter encounters a resident with serious environmental health concerns. All three of the resident's children are asthmatics. From the time the family was forced to seek residence in the shelter, the children—particularly the youngest—have had multiple, acute episodes of asthma. The shelter manager is unwilling to correct the building's problems of dust, mold,

and inadequate heating, and has in fact told residents that they will be evicted if they complain to the city about the conditions. There is a waiting list for the shelter, the only one available within the city limits. The mother sees no way out for herself and her children. Anxious and distraught, she asks the nurse for help.

On a *case advocacy* level, the nurse might empower client decision-making by providing information and support in the following ways (discussed further in Cary, 1992):

— set up an appointment with the mother to explore the situation further and provide support;

— give her "user friendly" information about causes and care measures for asthma, and answer her questions;

— get more information about the mother's financial status, legal status as a resident, her relationship with the shelter manager and other residents, and her abilities for decision making and autonomy;

— get more information about the shelter environment and the timing and intensity of the children's asthma episodes;

— based on the information discussed, help the client explore other housing options, make her aware of relevant supports such as legal aid organizations, and assist her in moving toward decision making to solve the problem;

— provide on-going encouragement as the mother attempts to implement her problem-solving plan.

In this example, let us say that the mother gains confidence and decides to discuss her concerns with the shelter manager. It becomes clear that no immediate changes are likely, but the mother is now more able to consider her other options realistically. She chooses to readjust her goals and moves to a group-home which is less conveniently located, but provides a healthier environment for her children.

So far, so good. But suppose the nurse, having helped this one family, becomes concerned that other families in the shelter may have similar problems. She may wonder how the manager gets away with providing substandard housing conditions that threaten his residents' health. She may wonder why a city of this size does not offer more than one shelter. Maybe she would like to see some publicly or privately financed programs to help homeless individuals and families make easier transitions from temporary shelters, group homes, and street living into permanent housing. This is where class advocacy at the policy level comes into the picture, as the nurse begins to act as a social change agent on behalf of a whole class of clients. What kind of advocacy strategies and techniques can she use for these aspects of the problem?

## STRATEGY OPTIONS

One particularly useful framework for conceptualizing advocacy strategies is a model formulated by Jack Rothman during the 1960s, at a time when many health and human service professionals were working with communities in controversial, quasi-political roles. Rothman (1968) outlined three very different types of policy advocacy (or "community organization practice"), which he termed *locality development, social planning,* and *social action.*

The first of these types, *locality development*, is appropriate where a high degree of consensus exists about a social problem. Here advocacy is a matter of mobilizing slack resources and energizing the interested parties around a common concern. An example of locality development would be a rural health nurse working with community residents and local organizations to monitor and safeguard the quality of local well water. A professional practicing this kind of advocacy needs skills in organizing, program development, communications and public speaking, coalition building, and mediation. The individuals and communities being helped are seen as clients, and the interactions between service providers and service recipients are warm and process-oriented. The effort is inclusive and cooperative. Any conflicts that arise are settled by empathetic understanding and compromise.

The second type, *social planning*, also presumes considerable consensus on the nature of the problem. This kind of advocacy effort tends to be highly technical—determining the optimal distribution of a scarce resource, or the most cost-effective technology for achieving an agreed-upon service outcome. The effort might well involve high-level inter-disciplinary collaboration with other health and human service professionals. For instance, nurses might be involved in a planning a program to address radon exposure in the community. Working with other technical experts, they would help plan and carry out surveys and epidemiologic studies to characterize the problem; design testing and remediation procedures; plan a risk communication strategy; and evaluate the intervention's effects. The skills needed emphasize scientific expertise, program planning, and evaluation research. In this kind of effort, those being helped are viewed as end consumers, who need to be consulted and kept informed but not necessarily involved in the technical details. The interactions among planners in this approach are usually task-oriented and somewhat impersonal. If conflicts should arise, they are (in theory) resolved rationally in the public interest, based on the best available expert opinion.

The third type, *social action*, applies to situations with strong disagreement over the nature of the problem, serious interest conflicts among the parties affected, and large power imbalances among different factions with a stake in the issue. Here value-based allegiances come into play, and advocacy activity is likely to become highly partisan, taking on the flavor of a crusade. An example would be a nurse who concludes that toxic emissions from a local industrial plant pose a danger to residents in a surrounding minority community, and need to be stopped. The nurse's next steps might include contacting appropriate regulatory agencies and persuading them to take urgent action; enlisting the aid of journalists to do an expose on the company's disregard for public health; advising community activists on how best to document the health damage; contacting and enlisting support from other health professionals; helping citizen groups explore legal action against the company; lobbying for stronger public policy on "environmental justice"; speaking at community meetings; and helping to organize rallies and protest demonstrations. In this kind of advocacy, experts come under pressure to take sides and to get actively involved in the tactics of power politics. Those being helped are seen as citizens asserting legitimate rights, and allies in a social justice cause. The effort is passionate, emotional, and often conspiratorial. Conflict is seen as inevitable and warfare metaphors are common.

Rothman's formulation underscores the important idea that policy advocacy can be done in various ways, all legitimate in their own terms. Health professionals often feel most comfortable staying within the social planning model, an advocacy role that maximizes their own technical contribution and does not involve them in activities that feel more like community politics. Locality development and social action styles of advocacy may seem unprofessional, counterproductive to problem solving, and possibly detrimental to one's career interests. But in reality, what can be accomplished through the planning approach alone is often fairly limited. In almost any environmental health problem, all three advocacy styles are likely to be relevant. For example, workers who have been occupationally exposed to carcinogenic chemicals will certainly benefit from medical surveillance, a social planning approach. But they may also need help with locality development efforts such as setting up support groups to deal with the emotional and family stress aspects of the problem, and social action advocacy to get the hazard abated and pursue their legal rights to compensation.

Another relevant construct is a typology of social change strategies formulated by Roland Warren (1963). He distinguishes among *collaborative* approaches (as in planning and advisory committees) in which citizens and authorities work cooperatively to reach an agreed-upon goal; *campaign* approaches (as in lobbying and public information) in which citizens act singly or collectively to persuade authorities that new problem definitions and solutions are needed; and *contest* strategies (as in picketing and protest marches) in which citizens organize to force attention to community problems that they feel are being ignored or mishandled by authorities.

The value of Warren's model lies in emphasizing that community concerns can take conflictual and troublesome forms and still represent a positive contribution toward problem solving. Being only human, nurses may feel tempted to "advocate" mainly with those who use collaborative approaches for problem solving, because interaction with them is comfortable and affirming. Those using campaign or contest strategies are easy to dismiss as unhelpful, obstructive, and irrational. But in environmental health issues, militant approaches may be seen by those immediately affected as necessary aspects of problem solving (Alinsky, 1989). Nurses' advocacy roles will need to connect with this reality.

It should be noted that both case advocacy and class advocacy involve some thorny ethical dilemmas (see Gilbert and Specht, 1976; Needleman and Needleman, 1974). For example, if the advocacy goals as defined by clients and communities differ sharply from the advocacy goals as defined by the nurse who is acting as advocate, what should happen? Also, advocacy may in principle be a poor way to allocate resources equitably within a social system, because the clients and issues with the most effective advocates will not necessarily be the same ones with the greatest need. But despite such unsettling second thoughts on an abstract level, the questions confronting nurses on the front line of practice remain immediate and compelling: how to help as much as possible with the human problems at hand. In relation to environmental health issues, the answers often lead in the direction of advocacy, particularly advocacy at the policy level.

## RESOURCES FOR BUILDING ADVOCACY SKILLS

At present, policy advocacy for structural change is not emphasized in nursing education, leaving nurses somewhat on their own for exploring strategy options and developing the necessary skills. Fortunately, a great many self-training guides and manuals are available for health and human service professionals interested in advocacy practice related to environmental health issues. Box F.1 below lists some good starting points.

Many resources also exist for particular skill areas. Box F.2 lists a small sample of the voluminous self-training literature available on the nuts and bolts of advocacy practice techniques such as lobbying, use of mass media, working with community groups, organizing, coalition-building, community research projects, giving expert testimony, and program development.

## NETWORKING WITH OTHERS

Finally, keep in mind that you don't have to work alone. Those interested in policy advocacy should get in touch with appropriate organizations and clearing houses, many of which can offer advice, moral support, and technical assistance as well as useful publications, slides, films, and speakers. Some particularly relevant organizations are listed in Box F-3.

For contact information on many similar organizations, see Appendix D of this report, and also these directories:

*The Directory of National Environmental Organizations,* St. Paul, Minnesota: U.S. Environmental Directories, 1988.

The U.S. Environmental Protection Agency, Office of Information Resources Management, *Information Resources Directory,* Fall 1989.

---

**Box F.1**
**Basic Bookshelf for Advocacy Practice at the Policy Level**
**Related to Environmental Health**

Bagwell, Marilyn and Sallee Clements. *A Political Handbook for Health Professionals.* Boston: Little, Brown and Company, 1985.

Legator, Marvin S. and Sabrina F. Strawn (eds.) *Chemical Alert! A Community Action Handbook.* Austin, TX: University of Texas Press, 1993.

Bobo, Kim; Jackie Kendall; Steve Max. *Organizing for Social Change: A Manual for Activists in the 1990's.* Cabin John, MD: Seven Locks Press, 1991.

Archer, S.E., and P.A. Goehner. *Nurses: A Political Force.* Monterey, CA: Wadsworth, Inc., 1982.

Stevens, K.R. (ed.). *Power and Influence: A Source Book for Nurses.* New York: John Wiley and Sons, Inc. 1983.

Anderson, E.T. and J. McFarlane. *Community as Partner: Theory and Practice in Nursing.* Philadelphia: J.B. Lippincott, 1995.

Ross, Donald K. and Ralph Nader. *A Public Citizen's Action Manual.* New York: Grossman Publishers, 1973.

Fisher, Roger and William Ury. *Getting to Yes: Negotiating Agreement Without Giving in.* New York: Penguin Books, 1981.

Wasserman, Gary. *The Basics of American Politics,* 3rd ed. Boston: Little, Brown and Company, 1982.

Hadden, Susan G. *A Citizen's Right to Know: Risk Communications and Public Policy.* Boulder, CO: Westview Press, 1989.

## Box F.2
## Additional Resources for Advocacy Practice at the Policy Level Related to Environmental Health

American Nurses Association. *Handbook for Political Media.* Washington, DC: American Nurses Association, undated.

American Association of University Women. *AAUW Community Action Tool Catalog: Techniques and Strategies for Successful Action Programs.* Washington, DC: AAUW Sales Office, 1981.

Amy, Douglas. *The Politics of Environmental Mediation.* New York: Columbia University Press, 1987.

Auvine, Brian et al. *A Manual for Group Facilitators.* Madison, WI: The Center for Conflict Resolution, 1985. Address orders to: New Society Publishers, P.O. Box 582, Santa Cruz, CA 95061-0582.

Avery, Michel. *Building United Judgment: A Handbook for Consensus Decision Making.* Madison, WI: The Center for Conflict Resolution, 1985. Address orders to: New Society Publishers, P.O. Box 582, Santa Cruz, CA 95061-0582.

Ballinger, Bruce and Adela Awner. *Membership Recruiting Manual.* Helena, MT: Northern Rockies Action Group, 1981. Address orders to: 9 Placer Street, Helena, MT 59601.

Biagi, Bob. *Working Together: A Manual for Helping Groups Work More Effectively.* Amherst, MA: Center for Organizational and Community Development, undated. Address orders to: 225 Furcolo Hall, University of Massachusetts, Amherst, MA 01003.

Bortin, Virginia. *Publicity for Volunteers: A Handbook.* New York: Walker and Company, 1981.

Boyte, Harry C. *Commonwealth: A Return to Citizen Action.* New York: The Free Press, 1989.

Brown, Cherie R. *The Art of Coalition Building: A Guide for Community Leaders.* New York: The American Jewish Committee, 1990. Address orders to: 165 East 56th Street, New York, NY 10022, 212-751-4000.

deKieffer, D. *How to Lobby Congress.* New York: Dodd, Mead & Co., 1981.

Draves, William A. *How to Teach Adults.* Manhattan, KA: The Learning Resources Network, 1984. Address orders to : 1554 Hayes Drive, Manhattan, KA 66502.

Gordon, Robbie. *We Interrupt This Program: A Citizen's Guide to Using the Media for Social Change.* Amherst, MA: Center for Organizational and Community Development, 1978. Address orders to: 225 Furcolo Hall, University of Massachusetts, Amherst, MA 01003.

Grimes, A.J. *A Guide for Providing Scientific Testimony.* Arlington, VA: The American Institute of Biological Sciences, 1977.

Ilich, J. and B. Jones. *Successful Negotiating Skills for Women.* Menlo Park, CA: Addison-Wesley Publishing Company, 1981.

Janeway, Elizabeth. *Powers of the Weak.* Morrow Quill Paperbacks, 1981.

Kalisch, G. J. and Kalisch, P. A. *Politics in Nursing.* Philadelphia: Lippincott, 1982.

Kretzmann, John P. and John L. McKnight. *Building Communities from the Inside Out.* Chicago: ACTA Publications, 1993. Address orders to: 4848 North Clark Street, Chicago, IL 60640.

Lester, et al. *Using Your Right to Know.* Arlington, VA: Citizens Clearinghouse for Hazardous Wastes, 1989.

Levey, Jane Freundel. *If You Want Air Time.* Washington, DC: National Association of Broadcasters, 1990. Address orders to: 1771 N Street, N.W., Washington, DC 20036.

O'Conner, John et al. *The Citizens Toxic Protection Manual.* Boston, MA: National Campaign Against Toxic Hazards, 1987.

Needleman, Herbert L. and Philip J. Landrigan. *Raising Children Toxic Free: How to Keep Your Child Safe from Lead, Asbestos, Pesticides, and Other Environmental Hazards.* New York: Farrar, Straus and Giroux, 1994.

Smith, D. *In Our Own Interest.* Seattle: Madrona Publishers, Inc., 1979.

Sparks, D. B. *The Dynamics of Effective Negotiation.* Houston, TX: Gulf Publishing Company, 1982.

Staples, Lee. *Roots to Power: A Manual for Grassroots Organizing.* New York: Praeger Press, 1984.

Taylor, Eleanor D. *From Issue to Action: An Advocacy Program Model.* Lancaster, PA: Eleanor D. Taylor, 1987. Address orders to: Family and Children's Service, 630 Janet Avenue, Lancaster, PA 17601.

Trapp, Shel. *Who, Me a Researcher? Yes You!* Chicago: National Training and Information Center, undated, $3.50. Address orders to: 810 N. Milwaukee Avenue, Chicago, IL 60622.

U.S. General Services Administration and U.S. Department of Justice. *Your Right to Federal Records: Questions and Answers on the Freedom of Information Act and the Privacy Act.* Washington, DC: USGSA & USDOJ, 1981. Address orders to: R. Woods, Consumer Information Center-N, P.O. Box 100, Pueblo, CO 81002.

Wilson, Marlene. *The Effective Management of Volunteer Programs.* Boulder, CO: Volunteer Management Associates, 1976. Address orders to: 320 South Cedar Brook Road, Boulder, CO 80302.

---

**Box F.3**
**Organizations Doing Policy Advocacy Related to**
**Environmental Health**

Nurses' Environmental Health Watch
181 Marshall Street
Duxbury, MA 02332

The Citizens Clearinghouse for Hazardous Wastes
P.O. Box 6806
Falls Church, VA 22040
703-237-2249

National Toxics Campaign
20 East Street, Suite 601
Boston, MA 02111
617-482-1477

Environmental Action
1525 New Hampshire Avenue NW
Washington, DC 20036

Environmental Defense Fund
257 Park Avenue S
New York, NY 10010
212-502-2100

---

**Box F.3  Continued**

Natural Resources Defense Council
40 West 20th Street
New York, NY 10011
212-727-2700

Center for Science in the Public Interest
1501 16th Street NW
Washington, DC 20036-1499
202-265-4954

The American Public Health Association
(especially section chairs for Environment, Occupational
Safety and Health, Public Health Nursing, and Social Work)
1015 15th Street, NW
Washington, DC 20005
Government Relations Office: 202-789-5650

Association of Occupational and Environmental Health Clinics
1010 Vermont Ave., NW, #513
Washington, DC 20005
202-347-4976 (national directory available)

The "COSH group" in your region
(These are union-based "Coalitions for Occupational Safety and Health"; national
directory available from NYCOSH, 275 Seventh Avenue, 8th Floor, New York, NY
10001; 212-627-3900)

---

# REFERENCES

Alinsky S. "Of Means and Ends," in *Rules for Radicals*. New York: Vintage Books, 1989.

Cary A. "Promoting continuity of care: Advocacy, discharge planning, and case management." Pp. 681–706 in Stanhope M and Lancaster J, *Community Health Nursing: Process and Practice for Promoting Health*. St. Louis, MO: Mosby Year Book, 1992.

Gadow S and Schroeder C. "An Advocacy Approach to Ethics and Community Health." Chapter 4 in Anderson ET and McFarlane J, *Community As Partner: Theory and Practice in Nursing*. Philadelphia: J.B. Lippincott, 1995 (in press).

Gilbert N and Specht H. "Advocacy and Professional Ethics." *Social Work*, 288–293, July 1976.

Kohnke MF. *Advocacy: Risk and Reality*. St. Louis: The CV Mosby Co., 1982.

Marks JH (ed). *Advocacy in Health Care*. Clifton, NJ: Humana Press, 1985.

Needleman M and Needleman C. *Guerrillas in the Bureaucracy: The Community Planning Experiment in the United States*. New York: John Wiley, 1974.

Nelson ML. Advocacy in nursing. *Nursing Outlook*, 36(3):136–141, 1988.

Rothman J. "Three Models of Community Organization Practice," from the proceedings of the 1968 National Conference on Social Welfare, *Social Work Practice 1968*. New York: Columbia University Press, 1968.

Warren RL. "A Community Model," pp. 9–20 in Warren RL, *The Community in America*. Chicago: Rand McNally & Company, 1963.

Winslow GR. "From loyalty to advocacy: A new metaphor for nursing." *Hastings Center Report*, 14 (6):32–40, 1984.

# G

# Taking an Exposure History

Appendix G provides two examples of environmental and occupational history-taking forms that could be used by nurses in a variety of practice settings. The first form, *Comprehensive Occupational and Environmental History*, was created for a faculty development workshop on Environmental and Occupational Health offered by the University of Maryland at Baltimore (June, 1993), the second, *Occupational and Environmental Health History Form*, is reprinted, with permission, from Alyce B. Tarcher's *Principles and Practice of Environmental Medicine* (Plenum Publishing Co., 1992). Both forms enable nurses and other health professionals to assess individual risk and the need for prevention, to diagnose and treat occupational and environmental illnesses, and to develop a sensitivity to the environmental conditions in a community that may contribute to ill health. Taking an exposure history also provides an opportunity for nurses to enhance their relationship with patients by learning more about an individual's workplace, home, and community environments.

# Comprehensive
# Occupational and Environmental History

## Work History

1. List your current and past longest held jobs, including the military:

| Company | Dates Employed | Job Title | Known Exposures |
|---------|----------------|-----------|-----------------|
| _____ | _____ | _____ | _____ |
| _____ | _____ | _____ | _____ |
| _____ | _____ | _____ | _____ |
| _____ | _____ | _____ | _____ |
| _____ | _____ | _____ | _____ |
| _____ | _____ | _____ | _____ |

2. Do you work full-time?   NO____   YES____   How many hours per week?____

3. Do you work part time?   NO____   YES____   How many yours per week?____

4. Please describe any health problems or injuries that you have experienced in connection with your present or past jobs:

5. Have you ever had to change jobs due to health problems or injuries?   YES____   NO____
   If so, describe:

   Did any of your co-workers experienced similar problems?

6. In what type of business do you currently work?

7. Describe your work (what do you actually do):

# Work History (continued)

8. Have you had any current or past exposure (through breathing or touching) to any of the following?

| | | | | | |
|---|---|---|---|---|---|
| __acids | __carbon | __dichlorobenzene | __manganese | __pesticides | __toluene |
| __alcohols | tetrachloride | __ethylene dibromide | __mercury | __phenol | __TDI or MDI |
| __alkalies | __chlorinated | __ethylene dichloride | __methylene | __phosgene | __trichloroethylene |
| __ammonia | napthalenes | __fiberglass | chloride | __radiation | __trinitrotoluene (TNT) |
| __arsenic | __chloroform | __halothane | __nickel | __rock dust | __vibration |
| __asbestos | __chloroprene | __heat (severe) | __noise (loud) | __silica powder | __vinyl chloride |
| __benzene | __chromates | __isocyanates | __PBBs | __solvents | __welding fumes |
| __beryllium | __coal dust | __ketones | __PCBs | __styrene | __x-rays |
| __cadmium | __cold (severe) | __lead | __perchloroethylene | | __talc |

9. Did you receive any safety training about these agents? YES___ NO____
   Explain:

10. Are you involved in any work processes such as grinding, welding, soldering, or polishing that create dust, mists, or fumes?     YES____     NO____     (If yes, describe):

11. Did you use any of the following personal protective equipment when exposed?
    ___boots              ___glasses/goggles          ___safety shoes    ___sleeves
    ___coveralls          ___gloves                   ___shield          ___welding mask
    ___earplugs/muffs     respirator

12. Is your work environment generally clean? If not, describe:

13. What ventilation systems are used in your workplace?

14. Do they seem to work? Are you aware of any chemical odors in your environment (if so, explain)?

15. Where do you eat, smoke, and take your breaks when you are on the job?

16. Do you use a uniform or have clothing that you wear only to work?

17. How is your work clothing laundered (at home, by employer, etc.)?

18. How often do you wash your hands at work and how do you wash them? (running water, special soaps, etc.)

19. Do you shower before leaving the worksite?

20. Do you have any physical symptoms associated with work? If yes, describe:

21. Are other workers similarly affected?

## Home Exposures

1. Which of the following do you have in your home?

___air conditioner ___electric stove ___woodstove ___central heating (gas or oil?)

___air purifier ___fireplace

2. In approximately what year was your home built? _____

3. Have there been any recent renovations? If yes, describe:

4. Have you recently installed new carpet, bought new furniture, or refinished existing furniture? If yes, explain:

5. Do you use pesticides around your home or garden? If yes, describe:

6. What household cleaners do you use? (List most common and any new products you use.)

7. List all hobbies done at your home:

Are any of the agents listed earlier for work exposures encountered in hobbies or recreational activities?

Is any special protective equipment or ventilation used during hobbies? Explain:

8. What are the occupations of other household members?

9. Do other household members have contact with any form of chemicals at work or during leisure activities? If so, explain:

10. Is anyone else in your home environment having symptoms similar to yours?
If yes, explain briefly:

## Community Exposures

1. Are any of the following located in your community?

    ___industrial plant      ___major source of air pollution      ___waste site

    ___landfill      ___toxic spill      ___other_____

2. What is your source of drinking water?

    ___private well      ___public water source      ___other_____

3. Are neighbors experiencing any health problems similar to yours? If yes, explain.

---

## Key Occupational and Environmental Health Questions to be asked with all histories

1.      What are your current and past, longest held jobs?

2.      Have you been exposed to any radiation or chemical liquids, dusts, mists, or fumes?

3.      Is there any relationship between current symptoms and activities at work or at home?

# Occupational and Environmental Health History Form

I. **IDENTIFICATION**

Name _____

Address _____

_____ Zip _____

Telephone: home _____ work _____

Soc. Sec. _____ - ___ - _____

Sex: M _____ F _____

Birthday _____

II. **OCCUPATIONAL HISTORY**

Fill in the table below listing all jobs at which you have worked, including short-term, seasonal, and part-time employment. Start with your present job and go back to the first. Use additional paper if necessary.

| Workplace (Employer's name and address or city) | Dates worked From | To | Type of Industry (Describe) | Your job duties (Describe) | Health hazards in workplace (Gases, dust, metals, solvents, radiation, infectious agents, etc.) | Protective equipment used (Describe) | Health problems related to work (Describe) |
|---|---|---|---|---|---|---|---|
|  |  |  |  |  |  |  |  |
|  |  |  |  |  |  |  |  |
|  |  |  |  |  |  |  |  |
|  |  |  |  |  |  |  |  |

## Occupational Exposure

1. Describe any health problems or injuries related to present or past jobs.

2. Have you or your coworkers had health problems or injuries?

3. Do you believe you have health problems related to your present or past work?

4. Have you been off of work because of a work-related illness or injury? If so, describe:

5. Have you worked with a substance that caused a skin rash? What was the substance? Describe your reaction.

6. Have you had trouble breathing, coughing, or wheezing while at work? If so, describe:

7. Do you have any allergies? If so, describe:

8. Have you had difficulty conceiving a child?

9. Do you have any children who were born with abnormalities?

10. Do you smoke or have you ever smoked cigarettes, cigars, or pipes? For how long and how many per day?

11. Do you smoke on the job?

12. Have you ever worked at a job or hobby in which you came into direct contact with any of the following substances through breathing, touching, or direct exposure? If so, please place a checkmark beside the substance.

| | |
|---|---|
| Acids | Halothane |
| Alcohols (industrial) | Heat (severe) |
| Alkalis | Isocyanates |
| Ammonia | Ketones |
| Arsenic | Lead |
| Asbestos | Manganese |
| Benzene | Mercury |
| Beryllium | Methylene chloride |
| Cadmium | Nickel |
| Carbon tetrachloride | Noise (loud) |
| Chlorinated naphathalenes | PBBs |
| Chloroform | PCBs |
| Chloroprene | Perchloroethylene |
| Chromates | Pesticides |
| Coal dust | Phenol |
| Cold (severe) | Phosgene |
| Dichlorobenzene | Radiation |
| Ethylene dibromide | Rock dust |
| Ethylene dichloride | Silica powder |
| Fiberglass | Solvents |

| | |
|---|---|
| Styrene | Trinitrotoluene |
| Talc | Vibration |
| Toluene | Vinyl chloride |
| TDI or MDI | Welding fumes |
| Trichloroethylene | X rays |

If you have answered "yes" to any of the above, please describe your exposure on a separate sheet of paper.

## Environmental Exposure

1. Do you live in the central city or in a rural, urban, or suburban area?

2. Have you ever changed your residence or home because of a health problem? If so, describe:

3. Do you live in the immediate vicinity of a refinery, smelter, factory, battery recycling plant, hazardous waste site, or other potential pollution source?

4. Do you (and your child) live in or regularly visit a building with peeling or chipped lead paint (e.g., built before 1960)? Has there been recent, ongoing, or planned renovation or remodeling of this structure(s)?

5. Do any members of your household have contact with dusts or chemicals in the workplace that are then brought into the home?

6. Do you have a hobby that you do at home? If so, describe:

7. Do you fumigate your home or use pesticides in and around your home and on a pet? Do you use mothballs?

8. What cleaning agents and solvents are used in your home?

9. Is there evidence of mold in your home?

10. Which of the following do you use in your home?

| | |
|---|---|
| Air conditioner | Humidifier |
| Electric stove | Wood stove |
| Air purifier | Gas stove |
| Fireplace | Unvented kerosene heater or gas heater |

11. What is your source of drinking water?

Community water system
Private well
Bottled water

# H

# Acknowledgments

The committee wishes to acknowledge and express its appreciation for the assistance and input provided by the following individuals:

Jacqueline Agnew, Ph.D.
Johns Hopkins School of Hygiene and Public Health

Laura Baird, M.S.
Institute of Medicine

Gershon Bergeisen, M.D., M.P.H.
U.S. Environmental Protection Agency

Patricia Bertsche, R.N., M.P.H.
Occupational Safety and Health Administration

Helen Ellis, R.N., B.S., C.O.H.N.
National Academy of Sciences

Lynda Firment, R.N.C., C.D.H.N.
U.S. Department of Energy

Beth Hibbs, R.N., M.P.H.
Agency for Toxic Substances and Disease Registry

Patricia Howard, R.N.
Senator Daniel Inouye's Office

Carole Hudgings, R.N., Ph.D.
Agency for Health Care Policy and Research

Honorable Daniel Inouye
U.S. Senate

Bernadine Kuchinski, Ph.D.
National Institute for Occupational Safety and Health

Nancy Lescavage, R.N.
Senator Daniel Inouye's Office

Jane Lipscomb, R.N., Ph.D.
National Institute for
    Occupational Safety and
    Health

Max Lum, Ph.D., M.P.A.
National Institute for
    Occupational Safety and
    Health

Diane Mancino, M.A., R.N.,
    C.A.E.
National Student Nurses
    Association

Patricia Moritz, Ph.D., R.N.,
    F.A.A.N.
National Institute of Nursing
    Research

Donna Orti, M.S.
Agency for Toxic Substances and
    Disease Registry

Gerald Poje, Ph.D.
National Institute of
    Environmental Health
    Sciences

David Rall, M.D., Ph.D.
National Institute of
    Environmental Health
    Sciences

Barbara Redman, R.N., Ph.D.,
    F.A.A.N.
American Nurses Association

Virginia Ruth, R.N., Dr.P.H.
University of Maryland at
    Baltimore

Marla Salmon, Sc.D., R.N.,
    F.A.A.N.
Health Resources and Services
    Administration

Anne Sassaman, Ph.D.
National Institute of
    Environmental Health
    Sciences

Barbara Sattler, R.N., Ph.D.
University of Maryland at
    Baltimore

Allene Scott, M.D.
University of Pittsburgh

Moira Shannon, Ed.D., M.S.N.,
    R.N.
Health Resources and Services
    Administration

Kenneth Shine, M.D.
Institute of Medicine

Jeannie Viges, R.N., B.S.N.
Occupational Safety and Health
    Administration

Ginger Wandless, B.A.
U.S. Environmental Protection
    Agency

Karen Worthington, M.S., B.S.,
    R.N.
American Nurses Association

Gooloo Wunderlich, Ph.D.
Institute of Medicine

# I

# Committee and Staff Biographies

## COMMITTEE

**LILLIAN H. MOOD** (*Chair*), R.N., M.P.H., F.A.A.N., is Director of Risk Communication, Environmental Quality Control, in the South Carolina Department of Health and Environmental Control. Formerly, she was Assistant Commissioner and State Director of Public Health Nursing for the South Carolina Department of Health and Environmental Control and is an adjunct professor at the University of South Carolina College of Nursing. She was on the Institute of Medicine committee studying the future of public health and has been honored as a fellow by the American Academy of Nursing and the W. K. Kellogg Foundation.

**ELIZABETH T. ANDERSON**, R.N., Dr.P.H., F.A.A.N., is Professor and Chair of the Department of Community Health and Gerontology at the University of Texas School of Nursing at Galveston. Dr. Anderson is also the director of the World Health Organization Collaborating Center in Nursing and Midwifery Development in Primary Health Care. She has written extensively on the role of community health nurses and the need for greater education and curriculum development in this area. She received the 1994 American Public Health Association's Public Health Nursing Creative Achievement Award. She serves on the editorial advisory boards of *Advances in Nursing Science* and *Public Health Nursing*.

**HENRY A. ANDERSON**, M.D., is Chief Medical Officer for Occupational and Environmental Health for the Wisconsin Division of Health.

He is also a State Epidemiologist for Wisconsin, an Adjunct Professor at the University of Wisconsin, and a Lecturer for the Department of Community Medicine at Mount Sinai School of Medicine, New York City. As a leading advocate for the State of Wisconsin on health, Dr. Anderson has written extensively on a broad spectrum of issues including childhood lead exposures, cigarette smoking, occupational illness, asbestos disease, public health surveillance, and risk management. Dr. Anderson is currently Associate Editor of the *American Journal of Industrial Medicine* and an editorial board member for *Health and Environmental Digest*.

**NORMAN DEPAUL BROWN**, R.N., Ed.D., is an Associate Professor at the College of Nursing at the University of Arkansas, where he is responsible for curriculum development and teaching both undergraduate and graduate programs. Dr. Brown has been a principal investigator on several projects focusing on health reform and community health practice, while also authoring publications on barriers to faculty practice and current administrative practice and management in academic nursing centers. In addition, in 1993, Dr. Brown was appointed as a third-year fellow for the U.S. Public Health Service's Primary Care Fellowship, cosponsored by the Agency for Health Care Policy and Research.

**GAIL F. BUCKLER**, R.N., M.P.H., C.O.H.N., is a Clinical Instructor at the University of Medicine and Dentistry of New Jersey's (UMDNJ)-Robert Wood Johnson Medical School in the Department of Environmental and Community Medicine and the Environmental and Occupational Health Sciences Institute (EOHSI), which is jointly sponsored by the UMDNJ-Robert Wood Johnson Medical School and Rutgers, the State University of New Jersey, She is also an Assistant Professor of Clinical Nursing at the UMDNJ-School of Nursing, where she is Director of the Occupational Health Nursing Program. As a clinical occupational health nurse, Ms. Buckler has published several articles on occupational hazards, quality assurance audits of medical surveillance programs, and indoor air quality.

**ANN H. CARY**, Ph.D., M.P.H., R.N., is a Professor and Associate Dean at the Louisiana State University Medical Center School of Nursing. Dr. Cary received a B.S. in nursing from Louisiana State University, an M.P.H. from Tulane University, and a Ph.D. in education and counseling from Catholic University. She serves on the Nursing Intervention Payment Panel for the American Nurses Association (ANA) and is Chair for the ANA Council of Professional Nursing Education and Development. Dr. Cary is Past-President of the Association of Community Health Nursing Educators, active in the American Public Health Association, was to the U.S. Public Health Service (USPHS) Public Health Study Group, and is a Primary Care Fellow with the USPHS. She has published in the areas of environmental health, credentialing case management, community health nursing, home health care, and interdisciplinary collaboration.

**SUE K. DONALDSON**, Ph.D., R.N., F.A.A.N., is Dean of the School of Nursing at Johns Hopkins University. Before coming to Johns Hopkins, Dr. Donaldson was a Professor in the Department of Physiology at the School of Medicine, a Professor and Chair of Nursing Research, and Director of the Research Center for Long Term Care of the Elderly at the University of Minnesota. She continues to act as a consultant to the National Institute for Nursing Research and to universities around the country. Dr. Donaldson is a pioneer in nursing research, having been the principal investigator for the National Institutes of Health on basic science and nursing research through grants since 1974. In 1992, Dr. Donaldson was inducted as a Fellow of the American Academy of Nursing. Dr. Donaldson is also a member of the Institute of Medicine.

**GERALDENE FELTON**, Ed.D., R.N., F.A.A.N., is Professor and Dean of the College of Nursing at the University of Iowa. In 1990-1991, she served as the Chair of the Task Force on Membership for the American Academy of Nursing and President of the American Association of Colleges of Nursing. Dr. Felton's research and numerous publications have focused on mandating new initiatives for nursing education, perspectives on differentiated practice, the future of nursing research, and the biological rhythm phenomenon. Having been awarded numerous grants for her work in nursing leadership and practice, she is currently working on a grant from the U.S. Department of Health and Human Services to implement a nurse anesthetist education program.

**ELAINE L. LARSON**, Ph.D., M.A., R.N., is a Dean and Professor in the School of Nursing at Georgetown University. She is also on the Council of Deans, Hospital Executive Staff, Medical Center Council, and the Committee on Control of Hospital Infections at Georgetown Hospital. Prior to her move to Georgetown University, Dr. Larson served as Professor with tenure and the Director of the Center for Nursing Research at Johns Hopkins University. She is also a distinguished lecturer and author of several books and journal articles focusing on a broad spectrum of issues, including infection control, critical care nursing, and nursing research. Dr. Larson is also a member of the Institute of Medicine.

**CAROLYN NEEDLEMAN**, Ph.D., is a Professor of Social Work and Director of the Occupational and Environmental Health Program at Bryn

Mawr College. She has 20 years of experience in the analysis, development, and evaluation of community-based health and human service programs. She serves on the Action Board of the American Public Health Association and frequently provides technical assistance to federal agencies such as the National Institute of Environmental Health Sciences, the Occupational Safety and Health Administration, and the National Institute for Occupational Safety and Health. At present, she is principal investigator or consultant in several community-based research projects related to environmental health and risk communication.

**DOROTHY S. ODA**, R.N., D.N.Sc., F.A.A.N., is Professor and Chair of the Department of Mental Health, Community, and Administrative Nursing at the University of California at San Francisco. Dr. Oda has served as Chair and continues to be a member of the Publications Board for the American Public Health Association. She is a Fellow of the American Academy of Nursing and the American School Health Association. Most recently, Dr. Oda was awarded the Henrik Blum Award for Outstanding Achievement in Public Health by the California Public Health Association. Her research has focused on investigating the effect of public health nursing on client health behavior and status.

**RANDOLPH F. R. RASCH**, Ph.D., R.N., is an Assistant Professor in the School of Nursing, University of North Carolina at Chapel Hill. Dr. Rasch is also a consulting family nurse practitioner for the Health Care Center of the SAS Institute, Inc. He has been the principal investigator on several projects focusing on patterns of health in men, classification of nursing interventions, and health services quality assurance issues. His research and national presentations have also examined the case study method in clinical practice, the role of male nurses, as well as the recruitment and retention of minority nursing students.

**KATHLEEN M. REST**, Ph.D., M.P.A. is an Assistant Professor in the Occupational Health Program in the Department of Family and Community Medicine at the University of Massachusetts Medical Center and an Adjunct Assistant Professor at the University of Massachusetts School of Public Health. Dr. Rest has extensive experience in curriculum and faculty development in occupational and environmental medicine, having directed one of the first federally-funded programs in this area for primary care physicians. She is the recipient of a University of Massachusetts grant for innovation in medical education, and is a founding member of the Boston-based Consortium for Environmental Education in Medicine (CEEM). She served as a consultant on the IOM report *The Role of the Primary Care Physician in Occupational and Environmental Health*. Dr.

Rest's research interests focus on policy issues in occupational and environmental health.

   **BONNIE ROGERS**, Dr.P.H., C.O.H.N., F.A.A.N, is an Associate Professor of Nursing and Public Health and the Director of the Occupational Health Nursing Program at the University of North Carolina, Chapel Hill. Dr. Rogers served as Chair of the Institute of Medicine's workshop on Nursing and Occupational and Environmental Health and as a distinguished lecturer for Sigma Theta Tau International. Her research and publication activities include topics on risk assessment in nursing, the occupational hazards of health care workers, and ethics in occupational health nursing. Dr. Rogers recently authored (1994) *Occupational Health Nursing: Concepts and Practice*, which is the only textbook on the subject.

   **META A. SNYDER**, M.P.H., M.S., R.N., is formerly the Director of the National Center for Hazard Communication and the Deputy Director of the Environmental and Hazardous Materials Management Program at the University of Maryland. She is also a Faculty Associate at the University of Maryland School of Nursing and a group facilitator and resource person for the University of Maryland at Baltimore's (UMAB) School of Medicine on occupational/environmental health. Ms. Snyder serves as Chair for the Occupational Health Nursing Committee for the American Public Health Association and is on the Board of Directors for the Association of Occupational and Environmental Clinics. In addition, she has written and lectured extensively on the issues of risk communication and occupational and environmental health.

## STAFF

   **ANDREW M. POPE**, Ph.D., is a Senior Staff Officer and Study Director in the Institute of Medicine's Division of Health Promotion and Disease Prevention. His primary interests focus on occupational and environmental influences on human health, with expertise in physiology, toxicology, and epidemiology. Previously, in the Division of Pharmacology and Toxicology at the U.S. Food and Drug Administration, Dr. Pope's research focused on the neuroendocrine and reproductive effects of environmental substances on food-producing animals. During his tenure at the National Academy of Sciences, and since 1989 at the Institute of Medicine, Dr. Pope has directed and edited numerous reports on occupational and environmental issues; topics include injury control, disability prevention, biological markers, neurotoxicology, indoor allergens, and environmental medicine in the medical school curriculum.

**CARRIE E. INGALLS,** B.A., is a Research Assistant in the Institute of Medicine's Division of Health Promotion and Disease Prevention. Having graduated from the University of Richmond in 1993 with a degree in international studies, Ms. Ingalls is currently working on a her M.P.H. in health policy and program at the George Washington University. Her areas of concentration are epidemiology, environmental health, and oncology. Ms. Ingalls also worked for the Committee on Curriculum Development in Environmental Medicine at the Institute of Medicine before joining the Committee on Enhancing Environmental Health Content in Nursing Practice.

# Index